The Doctor's Book of Humorous Quotations

A Treasury of Quotes, Jokes, and One-Liners
About Doctors & Health Care

The Doctor's Book of Humorous Quotations

A Treasury of Quotes, Jokes, and One-Liners
About Doctors & Health Care

Compiled and Edited by

Howard J. Bennett, M.D.

Clinical Professor of Pediatrics
The George Washington University School of Medicine
and Health Sciences
Washington, D.C.

HANLEY & BELFUS, INC.
PHILADELPHIA, PA

Publisher: HANLEY & BELFUS, INC.
Medical Publishers
210 South 13th Street
Philadelphia, PA 19107
(215) 546-7293; 800-962-1892
FAX (215) 790-9330
Web site: http://www.hanleyandbelfus.com

Also by Howard J. Bennett

The Best of Medical Humor:
A Collection of Articles, Essays, Poetry & Letters
Published in the Medical Literature, 2nd edition

Library of Congress Cataloging-in-Publication Data

The doctor's book of humorous quotations / edited by Howard J. Bennett.
    p. ; cm.
    Includes index.
    ISBN 1-56053-452-4 (alk. paper)
    1. Medicine—Humor. 2. Medicine—Quotations, maxims, etc. I. Bennett, Howard J.
    [DNLM: 1. Medicine—Collected Works. 2. Medicine—Humor. WZ305 D637 2000]
R705.D63 2001
610'.2'07—dc21
                                                       00-058090

THE DOCTOR'S BOOK OF HUMOROUS QUOTATIONS   ISBN 1-56053-452-4

Last digit is the print number: 9 8 7 6 5 4 3 2 1

For Ryan and Molly

Contents

Acknowledgments

The first people to acknowledge when putting together a book of this sort are the hundreds of talented individuals, some of whom remain nameless, who created all of these marvelous jokes and witty sayings in the first place. Their clever and perceptive words say something about doctors and health care that is both illuminating and rich.

Since I do most of my writing at night and on weekends, the book had a fairly long gestation. And while I did most of the research myself, a number of people sent me material that added to both the scope and quality of the collection. I would like to thank Drs. Jim Buxbaum, Howard Fischer, Glenn Harquist, Clifford Kuhn, Ludwig Lettau, Robert Matz, Stu Silverstein, Alan Stone, and Edward Thompson for their help. I would also like to thank Kyle Watanabe, an eclectic system programmer, who has a better appreciation for medical humor than many of the doctors I know. I would like to give a special thanks to Dr. Mark DePaolis who has some of the best quotes in the book and whose funny and insightful books should be required reading for any docs who want to learn how to use a light touch with patients: "Trust Me, I'm a Doctor," "Are You a Real Doctor?" and "Get Well Sooner."

I would like to thank Cassandra Allen, the Head of Collection Access at the National Library of Medicine, who continues to make it easier for me to do my research at that marvelous institution. I would also like to thank Rosalie Maggio and Allen Klein for their helpful suggestions regarding the preparation of my manuscript and Elizabeth Bunsa at the American Medical Association for tracking down some information I needed to beef-up the index. Finally, I would like to thank my family for putting up with me when I descended into the basement to work on the book or had the nerve to edit the manuscript during bath time and other events so I could finish on schedule.

A Word About the Next Edition

Although I spent four years putting this collection together, I suspect there are a lot of medical quotes and jokes that I missed. Please send me any funny stuff you run into so I can review it for the next edition. If your material is selected, you will receive an acknowledgment in the book. Send your material to:

Howard J. Bennett, MD
c/o The Doctor's Book of Humorous Quotations
Hanley & Belfus, Inc.
210 South 13th Street
Philadelphia, PA 19107

Introduction

I'll never forget the first time I was introduced to the way quotes are used in medical settings. It was July of 1976, and I had just begun my first clinical clerkship as a third-year medical student. My fellow students and I were oriented to the medical service at 7:30 AM and started "work rounds" by nine. As we stopped by each room, we saw the patients briefly, reviewed pertinent physical findings and results from the day before, and then discussed what was planned for that day. Our senior resident ran the show. He queried the interns about what they thought was going on and helped them manage their patients efficiently. Phil was an amazing individual. He was brilliant, personable, and had an encyclopedic memory. He also talked in footnotes. Whenever Phil wanted to emphasize something, he quoted an article that supported his point of view. "Well," he'd say pausing for dramatic effect, "Peterson published a study on this subject in *The New England Journal of Medicine* about six months ago." Phil would then give the volume and page numbers for the article and glance at each of the students on the team. This glance meant he expected us to photocopy the article after rounds, read it, and be prepared to discuss it with him at any time during the next few days. So this was what my fellow students had meant by "quoting the literature." A daunting task to be sure, though slowly and inexorably, all trainees learn to master this rite of passage so it can be passed on to the next generation.

One of the most interesting things about Phil is that he did not limit himself to quoting references from medical journals. He knew how overwhelming the process of becoming a doctor was. He also knew the value of humor as a tool to relieve the stress of hospital training. So Phil was an expert with another type of quote: the medical one-liner. He used these quotes on rounds with the same skill and frequency that he quoted journal articles. He regaled us with lines like, "If you don't take a temperature, you won't find a fever," "There's no such thing as bowel function at the VA," and "The first thing to do at a code is to check your own pulse." For students and doctors, these lines are immediately funny. They're not funny because they make fun of patients. Rather, they take some aspect of medical life and turn it around so the anxiety created by the situation is attenuated by wit. For example, the comment about not taking temperatures is amusing because it's often difficult to evaluate patients with fever and many times it's just due to a virus that goes away on its own. So if you don't take a temperature, you'll never know you have a problem in the first place. Of course, fever can also be due to a serious illness, which is what creates the tension (and the humor) in the line. The second quote is a comment about a problem that's common in hospitalized patients, namely, good bowel habits. Patients at the VA (Veteran's Hospital) often have chronic conditions that require lengthy admissions. Anyone who's worked at a VA hospital knows how much effort it takes to keep patients "regular." What makes the quote funny is that doctors and nurses work so hard to remedy the problem, while the line suggests that no one at the VA has any bowel function at all. Concerning the last quote, anyone who's taken a course in CPR knows that the first thing you're supposed to do with an unconscious victim is to check his airway, breathing, and circulation. While a patient's airway is just as important in the hospital setting, our primary concern is whether the patient's heart has stopped. When doctors are called to cardiac arrests ("codes") there is always some initial anxiety about what happened even as efforts are made to quickly and efficiently resuscitate the patient. Doctors have to be cool headed at times like these and what the quote is really saying is, "Before you resuscitate a patient, make sure you're calm and that you know what you're doing." It's because of the anxiety a doctor can feel in this situation that the comment about taking your own pulse is funny. No one does it, of course, but it expresses instantly the anxiety one feels.

The lines that Phil used on rounds made us laugh because they took serious situations and turned them around for comic effect. To analyze Phil's behavior now, I realize that he was a proponent of what Freud called *gallows humor*—the use of humor as a coping mechanism in serious and life-threatening situations.[1] We all knew Phil was a terrific doctor and that he cared deeply about his patients. When he used humor, he was expressing a universal response to stress. Phil taught us a great deal about what it takes to be a good doctor: to read and analyze the medical literature, to practice good medicine, and to be able to laugh at yourself in order to stay sane in a serious and demanding profession. It's now been almost 25 years since I had my first lessons on how to be a good doctor, and I have followed the teachings of my early role models as closely as possible.

When I got the idea to put this book together, I thought about my first experiences in the hospital and the ways I have used humor with colleagues and patients over the years.[2-4] Phil did not actually write the quotes he used with us on rounds. They have been passed down over the years from doctor to doctor. When I began to work on the book, one of my goals was to collect as many of these lines as I could. So I began by searching the recesses of my mind to recall all of the quotes I heard during my training as a student and resident. After I exhausted my own supply of material, I queried my friends and colleagues to see what they remembered, and then I went to the medical literature to flesh out the rest. Along the way, I read as many collections of quotes, jokes, and one-liners as I could find. I also searched the internet and watched hours of TV to find additional material. What surprised me during this phase of my research was how many non-physicians have had something funny to say about medicine and health care over the years. Two of the classics in this area are quotes by Mark Twain and a comedian named Carrie Snow. Twain's line is, "Be careful about reading health books. You may die of a misprint." Snow's line is, "Going to a male gynecologist is like going to an auto mechanic who never owned a car." These lines are very funny and contain the same nuggets of wisdom that are present in medical one-liners. As I ran into more and more quotes by authors and comedians, I decided to include any material that poked fun at medical issues whether it was written by doctors or lay people. This not only broadened the scope of the book, but also gives medical professionals the chance to see themselves through other people's eyes.

One of the things about humor that's difficult to reconcile is that what's funny to one person may be insulting to another. Although I tried to keep offensive material out of the book, the line between wit and poor taste gets blurred at times. For example, is it acceptable to have quotes in the book about serious diseases? George Bernard Shaw once said, "Life does not cease to be funny when people die any more than it ceases to be serious when people laugh." In a similar vein, Will Rogers once said, "Everything is funny as long as it is happening to someone else." What these quotes imply is that something might be funny at another person's expense. One of the quotes in the book is about Alzheimer's Disease by the prolific physician writer, Mark DePaolis: "While most people don't have Alzheimer's, it's something that folks over 30 think about every time they misplace their car keys." This line is funny because most of us worry at least a little about this disease, either because we know someone afflicted with the condition or because we're concerned that it might lie in our own future. I also included a couple of jokes on Alzheimer's that poke some good-natured fun at the condition. Are these jokes offensive? They might be to some people, but I included them because the disease casts such a large shadow over our society. One of my parents had Alzheimer's, yet these jokes do not offend me. On the contrary, like all humor, the feeling I derive from this material frees me from the weight of the disease. It's like an existentialist thumbing his nose at the universe: "Yes, life is tough and unfair at times, but I can laugh at my imperfections and infirmities, and it makes me stronger to do so." In the end, I used a simple formula when making my selections—if the material made me laugh or evoked a smile of recognition, I included it in the book.

The book is organized alphabetically so readers can browse through the collection randomly or focus on topics of interest right away. Most of the subject headings are medical, i.e., Anatomy, Diagnosis, Procedures, Treatment, etc. Some of the headings are more general, however, such as Death, Family, Lawyers, Parenting, etc. Each of these general headings was selected because it had some medical connection. For example, the entries under Family are not disease oriented, but they will be of interest to providers who work in pediatrics, family practice, and internal medicine. I tried to be as specific as possible in the way subject headings are arranged, i.e., the entries on Gallbladders and Hernias are listed separately and not under the heading, Surgery. I have also included a fair amount of cross referencing throughout the book to make it easier to find additional topics of interest. For example, when looking through the section on Roundsmanship, you'll be prompted to check out the sections on Case Presentations, Diagnosis, Pearls, Pimping, PMDs, and Turfing. Most of the material is presented in the book once. Some of it is located in more than one section, however, because doing so makes the material more accessible to people with different interests.

I tried to determine the authorship for each of the quotes in the book. Unfortunately, many medical quotes are "classics" and the original author is unknown. Likewise, many of the quotes are written as someone's "law," so the full name of the author is still unavailable. In some cases, I listed the author as the person who first published the line, even though he or she may not be the individual who originally penned the quote. For example, I did my residency in the late 1970's when Samuel Shem published *The House of God*.[5] Dr. Shem's book contains a number of very funny lines, and I give him "credit" for many of them. On the other hand, I know Dr. Shem did not come up with all of the quotes in his book because we were using some of them before the novel came out. The best example of this is one of the lines I mentioned at the beginning of the introduction: "If you don't take a temperature, you won't find a fever." This quote is in Shem's book, but I ascribe it to Anonymous because I know its origins are much earlier. This is clearly a less than exact science, though I tried to be consistent within an admittedly flawed approach.

The material in the book comes from a wide variety of sources: medical journals, books, magazines, remarks made at conferences or on rounds, humor talks, lectures, TV shows, movies, standup comedy routines, and even lines specifically written for the collection. In most cases, I included a quote's source in the reference section at the back of the book. If a quote has not been previously published and was written by a friend or colleague, I listed the source as "Personal Communication." If I was unable to track down the primary source for a quote, I usually included a secondary source, i.e., another collection of quotes or one-liners. There are three situations where the source information is incomplete. First, I recalled many classic medical quotes from my own experience and the original source for these quotes is unknown. Second, I found a number of one-liners on TV or the internet and it was impossible to list a source in such cases. Finally, I wrote a number of quotes for the book myself and obviously there is no source for this material.

When I started the collection, I originally intended it for a medical audience: students, residents, nurses, allied health professionals, and doctors. Midway through my research, it became apparent that a wider range of people might enjoy the book. Consequently, lay people who have an interest in medicine or who interact with health care professionals on a regular basis should find the book useful. My main hope is that the book will provide a quick laugh or pick-me-up at the end of a busy day. But I also hope it will serve a larger purpose. Humor is a wonderful tool. It can reduce the tension we live with on a daily basis and can help us communicate better with colleagues, students, and patients. To that end, the material in the book can be used during lectures and hospital rounds, at conferences, and even for curbside consults. It can be shared with office staff and can be used by speakers who are looking for funny lines to spice up their presentations to medical professionals. Patients appreciate humor just like we do. Although some of the material in the book is technical, much of it will be accessible to the average person and can therefore be shared during clinical encounters. I maintain a Humor Board in my waiting room that is filled with quotes, jokes, cartoons, and one-liners. Although I don't monitor the Board on a daily basis, it's not uncommon for me to hear patients laugh out loud while they're waiting to be seen.

So sit back and enjoy the book. I had a lot of fun putting it together and hope you enjoy reading it.

Howard J. Bennett

REFERENCES

1. Robinson V: "Medical" humor as gallows humor. In Humor and the Health Professions: The Therapeutic Use of Humor in Health Care. Thorofare, NJ, Slack Inc., 1991, pp 85–98.
2. Bennett HJ: Humor in the medical literature. J Fam Pract 1995;40:334–336.
3. Bennett HJ: Using humor in the office setting: A pediatric perspective. J Fam Pract 1996;42:462–464.
4. Bennett HJ: The Best of Medical Humor: A Collection of Articles, Essays, Poetry & Letters Published in the Medical Literature. Philadelphia, Hanley & Belfus, 2nd ed, 1997.
5. Shem S: The House of God. New York, Dell Publishing, 1978.

A

~ ABSCESS ~

A woman and her husband interrupted their vacation to see a doctor. The woman said, "I want this boil lanced right away, and I don't want an anesthetic because I'm in a big hurry."

The doctor was quite impressed. "You certainly are a brave woman," he said. "Where is the boil?"

The woman turned to her husband and said, "Show the doctor your boil, dear."

~ ACADEMIA ~

Remember, you can publish *and* perish.   — *B. McKee* [196]

An ounce of pretension is worth a pound of manure.   — *Steven E. Clark* [92]

To err is human. To forgive is against departmental policy.   — *Anonymous* [201]

We are all replaceable, usually by people of lesser quality.
— *Mark Weissman, MD* [246]

The Chief is always right!   — *Anonymous* [94]

Instructors can take a point and explain it. Assistant professors can take a point and turn it into a lecture. Associate professors can take a point and turn it into a course. Professors can take a point and turn it into a career. Deans have forgotten the point.   — *Lee Reichman, MD* [254]

Life is short and vacations are shorter, but paperwork is eternal.
— *Howard Bennett, MD* [40]

Guidelines for Administrators:
• When in charge, ponder.
• When in trouble, delegate.
• When in doubt, mumble. — *James H. Boren* [322]

You can't teach an old dogma new tricks. — *Dorothy Parker* [116]

The Golden Rule of Academic Advancement: Do unto others as they would do unto you; only do it first. — *Anonymous* [201]

The phrase "memorable presidential address" has to be the ultimate oxymoron.
— *Lewis B. Sheiner, PhD* [280]

Scientists at Stanford Medical Center have come up with a new procedure to reduce pompous behavior in doctors. Although it's only been tested in academic physicians, the initial results are quite promising. According to the lead author, *cerebral liposuction* should be available to the general public within the next few years. — *Howard Bennett, MD* [48]

A newspaper ad for an academic physician:
We're a big, sprawling teaching hospital in a seedy part of town. We haven't matched in three years, and our Physician-in-Chief just quit to go to law school. Are you an academic doc who is ready to deal with motivational atrophy, turf battles, cost overruns, sneering, pimping, and the occasional food fight? If so, this could be the match of a lifetime.

How many Chairmen does it take to change a light bulb?
— Chairmen don't change light bulbs. However, if you do a feasibility study, they might put it in next year's budget.

(See also Attendings, Committees, Education, Lectures, Tenure, Writing & Publishing)

~ ACCIDENTS ~

A minor injury is one that happens to someone else. — *Anonymous* [94]

A study in Toronto showed that using cellular phones while driving quadrupled the risk of getting into an accident. On the plus side, 39% of the drivers said they used their phone to call an ambulance after the crash.

— *Ludwig Lettau, MD* [246]

A New York clothing manufacturer was hit by a car while crossing the street. As he lay on the ground in pain, a little old lady put his head in her lap and asked, "Are you comfortable?" He answered, "I make a living."

After a serious accident, a woman lay in a coma. Her worried husband stood at her bedside for days. One afternoon the nurse said reassuringly, "Well, at least age is on her side."

"She's not so young," replied the husband. "She's forty-five."

At this point, the patient moved slightly and murmured, "Forty-four."

(See also Emergencies, First Aid, Heimlich Maneuver)

~ ACUPUNCTURE ~

A friend of mine is into Voodoo Acupuncture. He doesn't have to see anybody. He'll just be walking down the street, and all of a sudden . . . "Ah!"

— *Steven Wright* [135]

I had acupuncture once. It didn't hurt. It didn't cost much. And it didn't work.

— *Ryan James, MD* [246]

I called my acupuncturist the other night because I had a splitting headache. He told me to stick two forks in my ear and call him in the morning.

(See also Chiropractors, Homeopathy)

~ ACUTE ~

Acute, adj. Something that occurs without warning. As in the pain one gets when approached by a drug rep at the end of a busy day.

— Howard Bennett, MD [46]

~ ADHESIVE TAPE ~

There are two kinds of adhesive tape—that which won't stay on and that which won't come off.

— Maria Telesco [302]

~ ADMINISTRATION ~

(See Hospital Administration)

~ ADOLESCENCE ~

There are three developmental stages in adolescent girls: pubarche, menarche, and anarchy.

— Howard Bennett, MD [48]

Since adolescents are too old to do the things kids do and not old enough to do the things adults do, they do things nobody else will do.

— Anonymous [268]

When children enter adolescence, one hunts for signs of health, is desperate for the smallest indication that the child's problems will never be important enough for a TV movie.

— Delia Ephron [122]

A teenager never opens his mouth when speaking except when there is food in it.

— David Guttman, MD [151]

Carol is fifteen, to put it mildly.

— Joan Hess [157]

Remember that as a teenager you are at the last stage in your life when you will be happy to hear that the phone is for you.   — *Fran Lebowitz* [189]

Adolescence *is* a disease.   — *Anonymous* [94]

Few things are more satisfying than seeing your children have teenagers of their own.   — *Doug Larson* [105]

Oh, to be only half as wonderful as my child thought I was when he was small, and only half as stupid as my teenager thinks I am now.   — *Rebecca Richards* [105]

Adolescence is schizophrenia with a good prognosis.
                                            — *Thomas L. Coleman, MD* [62]

Never lend your car to anyone to whom you have given birth.
                                            — *Erma Bombeck* [268]

When I was a boy of 14, my father was so ignorant I could hardly stand to have the old man around. But when I got to be 21, I was astonished at how much the old man had learned in seven years.   — *Mark Twain (attrib.)* [283]

There's nothing wrong with teenagers that reasoning with them won't aggravate.
                                            — *Anonymous* [135]

If Abraham's son had been a teenager, it wouldn't have been a sacrifice.
                                            — *Scott Spendlove* [75]

A teenage girl had been talking on the phone for about an hour and then hung up.
   "Gee," said her father, "that was short. You usually talk for two hours."
   "It was a wrong number," replied the girl.

(See also Sex Education)

~ ADOPTION ~

My sister was in labor for 36 hours. Ow! She got wheeled out of delivery, looked at me, and said, "Adopt."   — *Caroline Rhea* [67]

A teenage girl complains about her neighbor's obnoxious younger brother:
If you were my brother, I'd put myself up for adoption.
                                    — *"Honey, I Shrunk the Kids"* [160]

I want to adopt a child. Not a baby, one with a job.   — *Linda Herskovic* [163]

~ ADVICE ~

Free medical advice is worth exactly what you pay for it.   —*Anonymous* [94]

Two weeks ago I took care of a lady who had fallen. After I examined her swollen knee, I told her to go home, elevate it, and put ice on it. Twenty minutes later she called me on the phone: "I talked to Mabel, my maid, who thinks we ought to put heat on this knee." I told her, "You know, this morning at breakfast I was talking to my maid, Ruthie, and she said to put ice on it."
                                    — *Christian Ramsey, Jr, MD* [252]

I was preparing to leave the hospital when one of the doctors gave me some last minute instructions. He told me to wait two weeks before I had sex and six weeks before I drove a car. Or was it the other way around? I was still a little foggy and the entire discussion confused me, so I just promised him that I wouldn't have sex and drive at the same time and let it go at that.
                                    — *Lewis Grizzard* [323]

It's said that half of what we tell patients will no longer be true in five years. Then again, most patients don't listen to what we tell them anyway.
                                    — *Anonymous* [135]

A rule of thumb in the matter of medical advice is to take everything the doctor says with a grain of aspirin.   — *Goodman Ace* [62]

A man ran into his doctor at the hardware store. He stopped him and said, "Six weeks ago I saw you in the office. After the visit, you told me to go home, get into bed, and stay there until you called. But you never called."

"I didn't?" the doctor said. "Then what are you doing out of bed?"

A doctor finally got to his table after breaking away from a patient who sought his advice for a medical problem.

"Do you think I should send her a bill?" the doctor asked a lawyer who was sitting next to him.

"Why not?" the lawyer said. "You rendered professional services by giving advice."

"Thanks," the doctor said. "I think I'll do just that."

When the doctor went to his office the following day, he found a note from the lawyer. It read, "For legal services, $50."

An old man visited his doctor for a swollen ankle and was given specific instructions as to what he should and shouldn't do. Shaking his head, he started to leave the office when the doctor said, "Hey, wait a minute, you forgot to pay me."

"Pay you for what?"

"For my medical advice."

"Hell no! I ain't gonna take it."

A doctor looked at the test results for one of his middle-aged patients and was greatly disturbed by what he saw. The man's cholesterol was off the chart, his blood pressure was close to stroke level, and his diabetes was raging out of control. He picked up the phone and called the patient's wife. "I just got your husband's tests back, but I need to speak with you before I give him the results. Your husband is a very sick man and unless you do exactly what I advise, he'll be dead in six months."

"What can I do, doctor?" the woman asked.

"You must remove all sources of stress from his life," the doctor said. "You have to keep the house spotlessly clean, you've got to cook him a nutritious meal three times a day, and you need to have sex with him whenever he asks."

The woman hung up the phone and turned to her husband. "That was Dr. Cama with your lab results," she said.

"What did he say?"

"He says you're gonna die."

The doctor said to his patient, "Look, Mr. Cohen, the best thing for you is to stop smoking, stop drinking, and cut down on all those fattening foods."

"Well, doc," Mr. Cohen said. "What's second best?"

"You seem to be recovering nicely," the doctor said. "These x-rays show some damage to the bone, but I wouldn't worry about it."

The patient said, "If your bones were damaged, I wouldn't worry about it either."

(See also Compliance, Patients & Patient Care, Second Opinions)

~ AGING ~

(See Old Age)

~ ALCOHOL ~

Even though a number of people have tried, no one has yet found a way to drink for a living. — *Jean Kerr* [173]

An alcoholic is someone who drinks more than his own doctor.
— *Anonymous* [94]

The superego is that part of the personality that is soluble in alcohol.
— *Harold Lasswell, Ph.D.* [247]

If you resolve to give up smoking, drinking and loving, you don't actually live longer, it just seems that way. — *Anonymous* [103]

There are more old drunkards than old doctors. — *Francois Rabelais* [99]

One tequila, two tequila, three tequila, floor. — *Dennis Miller* [135]

Health—what my friends are always drinking to before they fall down.
— *Phyllis Diller* [310]

Alcoholism isn't a spectator sport. Eventually the whole family gets to play.

— *Joyce Rebeta-Burditt* [(253)]

If you drink, don't drive. Don't even putt. — *Dean Martin* [(321)]

One reason I don't drink is that I want to know when I'm having a good time.

— *Nancy Astor* [(17)]

I have cerebral palsy, and I don't understand why people will go out of their way to drink so they walk like me. — *Geri Jewell* [(311)]

A woman said to me, "Is it true that you still go out with young girls?" I said, "Yes, it's true." She said, "It is true that you still smoke 15 cigars a day?" I said, "Yes, it's true." She said, "It is true that you still take a few drinks a day?" I said, "Yes, it's true." She said, "What does your doctor say?" I said, "He's dead."

— *George Burns* [(106)]

Frank Burns: Margaret, I should warn you that alcohol is quite fattening.
Hot Lips Houlihan: That's alright Frank, I plan on throwing up later.

— *"M*A*S*H"* [(200)]

After a detailed examination of a recently admitted patient, the resident stated that he couldn't find the cause of the man's complaint, but added that it was probably due to heavy drinking.

"That's alright," the patient said. "Why don't you come back when you're sober?"

(See also Kidneys)

~ ALLERGY ~

To sneeze or not to sneeze, that is the question. — *E. L. Dimmick, MD* [(113)]

Never go to an allergist who has a stuffy nose. — *Molly Ryan, MD* [(246)]

On over-the-counter allergy medication:
These pills work very well to relieve symptoms, including the symptoms of awareness and conscious thought. — *Mark DePaolis, MD* [108]

Urticaria, n. Indicative of a desire to be manually transported by a third person; as, "The only reason that kid is screaming at her mother is that she wants urticaria." — *H. S. Grannatt* [145]

Little Miss Muffet (with a milk allergy)

Little Miss Muffet
Sat on a tuffet,
Eating her curds and whey;
She anaphylaxed,
Turned blue and collapsed,
And the ambulance whisked her away. — *Howard Bennett, MD* [45]

My allergy tests suggest that I may have been intended for some other planet. — *Walt Wetterberg* [196]

The reason I know I don't have allergies is that I don't believe in them. I just can't accept that the human body, which routinely manufactures things like parathyroid hormone from scratch, can be unable to control its own nasal passages when spring comes. — *Mark DePaolis, MD* [108]

We've made great medical progress in the last generation. What used to be merely an itch is now an allergy. — *Anonymous* [103]

Bloopers & Malapropisms:
• Mr. Cain reported an acute *exasperation* in his asthma. (exacerbation)
• A 68-year-old asthmatic presented to the emergency room with wheezing and shortness of *breast*. (breath)
• Past medical history reveals that the patient is sensitive to *macro lies*. (macrolides)
• Over the past two months, the patient reports a worsening of his *ectopic* dermatitis. (atopic)

A well-known allergist was scheduled to give Grand Rounds at a local hospital. As he was about to leave, his secretary said, "Dr. Keating, I've heard this lecture so many times, I bet I could do it myself. Why don't you rest at the back of the auditorium while I give the talk?"

Since the doctor had been up all night with a sick patient, he agreed.

At the hospital, the allergist settled into the back row for a nap while his secretary gave the lecture. At the end of the talk, the secretary asked if there were any questions.

"Yes," said one doctor, who proceeded to ask a rather difficult question.

The secretary got nervous, but recovered quickly and said, "That's such an easy question, I'm going to let my secretary answer it."

(See also Asthma)

~ ALTERNATIVE MEDICINE ~

(See Acupuncture, Chiropractors, Homeopathy)

~ ALZHEIMER'S DISEASE ~

While most people don't have Alzheimer's, it is something that folks over 30 think about every time they misplace their car keys.   — *Mark DePaolis, MD* [108]

A man goes to see his doctor for a checkup. After some tests, the doctor comes back with a serious look on his face. "I have some bad news and some really bad news," he says.

"Well, give me the really bad news first," the patient says.

"You have cancer and only six months to live."

"And the bad news?"

"You have Alzheimer's Disease."

"Thank God," the patient says. "I was afraid I had cancer."

What's the best thing about Alzheimer's disease?
— You keep meeting new friends.

What's the second best thing about Alzheimer's disease?
— You never have to watch reruns on TV.

(See also Memory, Old Age)

~ AMERICAN MEDICAL ASSOCIATION ~

There are a lot of doctors who don't belong to the AMA. Some think it's an elitist group that only cares about making money. Others, like myself, refuse to join any group that doesn't have a secret decoder ring.

— *Mark DePaolis, MD* [108]

~ AMNESIA ~

Right now, I'm having amnesia and déjà vu at the same time. I think I've forgotten this before.
— *Steven Wright* [194]

Amnesia: The condition that enables a woman who has gone through labor to have sex again.
— *Joyce Armor* [13]

(See also Memory)

~ ANATOMY ~

Gross anatomy will dominate your life during the freshman year of medical school, for better or worse. Usually for worse.
— *Anne Eva Ricks, MD* [256]

Anatomy is something everyone has, but it looks better on a girl.
— *Bruce Raeburn* [71]

Advice to first year medical students:
In anatomy it is better to have learned and lost than never to have learned at all.
— *W. Somerset Maugham* [205]

"Miss Ryan," said the anatomy teacher, "would you please tell the class what part of the body enlarges to five times its normal size during periods of agitation or emotional excitement?"

Blushing, the woman said, "Professor, I would rather not answer that question."

Raising an eyebrow, the professor asked, "Oh? And why not?"

"Well, sir, it's kind of personal."

"Not at all," he blustered. "The correct answer is the pupil of the eye, and your response tells me two things. First, you didn't read last night's assignment. And second, marriage is going to leave you a tremendously disappointed young woman."

(See also Body, Cadavers)

~ ANEMIA ~

(See Iron Deficiency)

~ ANESTHESIA ~

When in doubt, blame the surgeon.
— *Anonymous* [94]

On the common belief that anesthesiologists are dull individuals:
Contrary to popular belief, they do more than just talk you to sleep—some of them actually use drugs.
— *Anne Eva Ricks, MD* [256]

An epidural is a needle you put in a woman's back that makes her numb from the waist down . . . for years.
— *Chip Franklin* [135]

Law of Local Anesthesia: Never say "Oops!" in the operating room.
— *Anonymous* [203]

I had general anesthesia recently. It's so weird. You go to sleep in one room and then you wake up four hours later in a totally different room. Just like college.

— *Ross Shafer* [96]

Mr. Anesthetist, if the patient can keep awake, surely you can.

— *Wilfred Trotter* [298]

Bloopers & Malapropisms:
• The patient was *excavated* in the operating room. (extubated)
• Surgery was performed under General *Anastasia*. (anesthesia)

When a businessman got his bill for gallbladder surgery, he was shocked at the anesthesiology fee. He wrote a letter to the anesthesiologist asking him how he could justify $800 for a procedure that lasted only an hour and a half. The doctor sent the man a brief note that read: "It costs $50 to put you to sleep. The other $750 is to make sure you wake up. Most patients prefer the whole package."

A surgeon was discussing an upcoming operation with one of his wealthy patients.
    "Would you prefer a local anesthetic?" he inquired.
    "I can afford the best," replied the patient. "Get me something imported."

How many anesthesiologists does it take to change a light bulb?
—Two. One to have a cup of coffee and the other to tell the surgeon he's taking too long to do it.

A lawyer was attempting to lighten his cross-examination of an anesthesiologist who was a plaintiff in a malpractice case.
    "I guess that means you and I are in the same business because we both put people to sleep," the lawyer joked.
    "Yes," replied the doctor, "but I wake them up."

(See also Surgery)

~ Antibiotics ~

Everybody knows that doctors make lousy patients. Psychiatrists are the worst. One of my psychiatrist dads called me last week to ask why his 5-year-old still had a fever on the third day of a cold. He put her on amoxicillin and was puzzled that she wasn't any better. I said, "Look, Jim, I don't put my kids on Prozac just because they're in a bad mood."
— *Rick Stevens, MD* [246]

Patients can get well without antibiotics.
— *Anonymous* [94]

On the field of Behavioral Bacteriology:
It would be beneficial for patients to know that the medicine being taken is not only killing an infecting microorganism, but that it is also making those organisms suffer.
— *Bruce K. Rubin, MD* [270]

A brief history of antibiotics:
  500 B.C. — Here, eat this root.
1000 A.D. — That root is heathen, say this prayer.
1400 A.D. — That prayer is superstitious, apply this leech.
1850 A.D. — That leech is barbaric, take this potion.
1900 A.D. — That potion is snake oil, swallow this pill.
1950 A.D. — That pill is ineffective, take this antibiotic.
2000 A.D. — That antibiotic is artificial, eat this root.

(See also Cephalosporins)

~ Anxiety ~

What, me worry?
— *Alfred E. Neuman* [230]

I once treated a patient who was so guilt ridden, he had "my fault" auto insurance.
— *Clifford Kuhn, MD* [246]

My grandfather was a Jewish juggler. He used to worry about six things at once.

— *Richard Lewis* [67]

Dr. Hartley: What do you do when you're upset?
Patient: Well, I've got a method that always works. I go into a dark room, open up the windows, take off all my clothes, and eat something cold. No, wait a minute, I do that when I'm overheated. When I have a problem I just go to pieces.

— *"The Bob Newhart Show"* [57]

I have low self-esteem. When we were in bed together, I would fantasize that I was someone else.

— *Richard Lewis* [84]

I have a new philosophy. I'm only going to dread one day at a time.

— *Charles M. Schultz, "Charlie Brown"* [96]

What's the difference between anxiety and panic?
— Anxiety is the first time you can't do it a second time. Panic is the second time you can't do it the first time.

(See also Neurotics, Phobias, Stress)

~ APHORISMS ~

• Where there's a pill, there's a way.
• Half a nurse is better than none.
• Every ward has a silver lining.
• Don't count your subjects until they're batched.
• A watched tot never soils.
• Traction speaks louder than words.
• A CAT scan a day keeps the lawyers away.

— *Howard Bennett, MD* [48]

(See also Hippocrates, Murphy's Laws)

~ Appendix ~

Cleve Ward's Maneuver: If the patient has right lower quadrant pain and no appendectomy scar, put one there. [248]

It's not true that the appendix is worthless—it has put thousands of surgeons in expensive cars.   — *Anonymous* [124]

The only time a man ever took anything from me was when my appendix was removed—and then he had to use chloroform.   — *Peggy Hopkins Joyce* [124]

Humans can survive easily without an appendix, but surgeons can do so only with difficulty.   — *Rudolf Virchow (attrib.)* [194]

~ Appointments ~

There are two types of services in our society—those that require an appointment and those where you wait in line. Then there are doctor's visits, where you get to do both.   — *Howard Bennett, MD* [48]

(See also Medical Practice)

~ Arteries ~

A man is as old as his arteries.   — *Thomas Sydenham* [298]

~ Arthritis ~

After a certain age, if you don't wake up aching in every joint, you're probably dead.   — *Tommy Mein* [184]

Life begins at forty, but so does arthritis. — *Sam Levenson* [242]

It was recently reported that sex is good for people with arthritis—it's just not that pleasant to watch. — *Jay Leno* [307]

The receptionist called one of Dr. Cama's patients.

"Mr. White, the check you gave us for your office visit came back."

"Then we're even," Mr. White said. "So did my arthritis."

An elderly woman goes to see a rheumatologist because she was having pain in her right knee. After examining his patient, the doctor says, "Well, Mrs. Wilson, you've got to understand that at your age, you're bound to have some pain in your joints."

"But doctor," she says, "my left knee is just as old as my right one and it doesn't hurt a bit."

A third year medical student began doing a history and physical on an elderly man.

"Tell me," asked the student, "do you suffer from arthritis?"

"Of course," snarled the old man. "What else can I do with it?"

(See also Gout, Knees, Lyme Disease, Orthopedics, Rheumatology)

~ ARTIFICIAL INSEMINATION ~

Artificial insemination—that's a scary concept. You know why? I don't want to have coffee with a stranger, let alone have his child. — *Rosie O'Donnell* [67]

Artificial insemination can be defined as copulation without representation. — *Anonymous* [269]

(See also Infertility)

~ Art of Medicine ~

What to say to patients when things aren't going as planned:
Medicine is an art, not a science. — *Anne Eva Ricks, MD* [255]

On practicing the Art of Medicine:
Look wise, say nothing, and grunt. — *William Osler, MD* [125]

When physicians talk about the "art of medicine" they usually mean healing, coping with uncertainty, or calculating their federal income taxes.
— *Frederick L. Brancati, MD* [63]

The Art of Medicine consists of amusing the patient while nature cures the disease. — *Voltaire* [103]

~ Aspirin ~

An aspirin a day keeps the cardiologist away. — *Mark DePaolis, MD* [109]

A rule of thumb in the matter of medical advice is to take everything the doctor says with a grain of aspirin. — *Goodman Ace* [62]

~ Asthma ~

My sister didn't have such a good day. She has asthma, and in the middle of an attack she got an obscene phone call. The guy said, "Did I call you or did you call me?" — *John Mendoza* [96]

Asthma is a disease that has practically the same symptoms as passion except that with asthma it lasts longer. — *Anonymous* [135]

(See also Allergy, Cough, Lungs)

~ ATROPHY ~

Atrophy, adj. To become smaller with disuse. As in the state of mind brought on by successfully matching in the residency of ones choice.

— *Howard Bennett, MD* [46]

~ ATTENDINGS ~

You know you're an attending when:
• You give advice more than you ask for it.
• You sit on more committees than you have letters in your name.
• The nurses expect you to bring the donuts.   — *Howard Bennett, MD* [40]

Attending's Motto: I may have my faults, but being wrong isn't one of them.

— *Anonymous* [203]

There are two rules that all medical students must learn:
• Rule #1. The attending is always right.
• Rule #2. Don't forget Rule #1.   — *Howard Bennett, MD* [40]

How many medical students does it take to change a light bulb?
— Three. One to hold the bulb, one to read the manual, and one to call the attending when it won't come out.

How many attendings does it take to change a light bulb?
— None. That's what medical students are for.

(See also Pearls, Pimping, PMDs, Roundsmanship)

~ AUTOPSY ~

From a courtroom transcript:

Q: Doctor, did you check for a pulse before you performed the autopsy?

A: No.

Q: Did you check the blood pressure?

A: No.

Q: So then, it is possible that the patient was still alive when you began the autopsy?

A: No.

Q: How can you be sure, Doctor?

A: Because his brain was sitting on my desk in a jar.

Q: But could the patient have still been alive nonetheless?

A: Only if he was a lawyer.

Q: Doctor, how many autopsies have you performed on dead people?

A: All of my autopsies have been performed on dead people.

(See also Pathology)

ℬ

~ BABIES ~

It sometimes happens, even in the best of families, that a baby is born. This is not necessarily a cause for alarm. The important thing is to keep your wits about you and borrow some money.   *— Elinor Goulding Smith* [289]

Never trust a naked baby.   *— Anonymous* [94]

Most people make babies out to be very complicated, but the truth is they have only three moods:
• Mood One: Just about to cry.
• Mood Two: Crying.
• Mood Three: Just finished crying.   *— Dave Barry* [24]

We've begun to long for the pitter-patter of little feet—so we bought a dog. Well, it's cheaper, and you get more feet.   *— Rita Rudner* [271]

Now the thing about having a baby—and I can't be the first person to have noticed this—is that thereafter you "have" it.   *— Jean Kerr* [172]

A baby is an alimentary canal at one end and no sense of responsibility at the other.   *— Anonymous* [135]

Super Babies are similar to regular babies except they belong to you.
                    — P. J. O'Rourke [135]

Keeping a baby requires a good deal of time, effort, and equipment, so unless you are prepared for this, we recommend that you start with a hamster, whose wants are far easier.   *— Elinor Goulding Smith* [289]

Out of the mouths of babes—usually when you've got your best suit on.
                    — G. Baxter [68]

Two women were talking about how their lives had changed in their first few months of motherhood. One of them said to the other, "How do you feel about sex after the baby?"

Her friend said, "Fine, just don't wake me."

(See also Adoption, Biologic Clock, Breast Feeding, Children, Diapers, Fatherhood, Motherhood, Parenting)

~ BACKACHE ~

A backache is man's greatest labor-saving device. — *Anonymous* [249]

I'm at an age when my back goes out more than I do. — *Phyllis Diller* [112]

(See also Chiropractor)

~ BACTERIA ~

Bacteria, n. Really, really tiny microorganisms. Doctors talk about them all the time, but frankly, we're not even sure they exist.
— *George Thomas, MD & Lee Schreiner, MD* [303]

Microbiologists rename their bugs every 10 years just to keep ahead of clinicians.
— *Rip Pfeiffer, MD* [248]

Microbes will always have the last word. — *Louis Pasteur (Attrib.)* [135]

How many microbiologists does it take to change a light bulb?
—Three. One to change the bulb and two to reclassify the bulb's genus and species name.

~ BALDNESS ~

A hair in the head is worth two in the brush.   — *Oliver Herford* [125]

One of the ironies of middle age is that as your waist gets thicker your hair gets thinner.   — *Howard Bennett, MD* [48]

Politically correct terms for baldness: scalp-impaired, follicularly challenged.
                                                       — *Anonymous* [135]

It is better to give than to recede.   — *Harry Crane* [104]

The only thing that can stop hair from falling is the floor.   — *Will Rogers* [88]

Babies haven't any hair.
Old men's heads are just as bare.
From the cradle to the grave,
Lies a haircut and a shave.   — *Samuel Hoffenstein* [298]

There are three ways in which a man can wear his hair: parted, unparted, departed.   — *Anonymous* [65]

If a man is bald in front, he's a thinker. If he's bald in back, he's a lover. If he's bald in front and back, he thinks he's a lover.

~ BEDSIDE MANNER ~

Your bedside manner is admirable, Doctor. I'm sure your patients recover quickly just to get away from you.   — *"Q" to Dr. Beverly Crusher* [295]

(See also Doctor-Patient Communication)

~ BEDWETTING ~

I slept in the same bed with six brothers. We had a bed wetter. It took us three years to figure out who it was.   — *Bob Hope* [243]

Two eight year old girls met after school to talk about their upcoming spring break.

"Why don't you come to the beach with me and my family?" one of them asked.

"I'd like to," said her friend, "but I wet the bed at night so I'm nervous about taking trips with my friends."

"How often do you wet the bed?" the first girl asked.

"About once a week."

"That's simple," her friend answered. "Just wet your bed the night before we leave."

~ BEEPERS ~

Ratner's Law: Beepers work better if you turn them on. [135]

I don't like beepers. If I have strange noises coming from my body unexpectedly, I want it to mean I have indigestion.   — *Gene Perret* [244]

(See also Night Call)

~ BEHAVIOR MANAGEMENT ~

The Laws of Behavior Modification only apply to other people's children.
                    — *Lawrence G. Calhoun, Ph.D.* [80]

~ BILLS ~

Beware of patients who call you "Doc." They rarely pay their bills.
                    — *William Osler, MD (attrib.)* [141]

At a recent party, a tipsy man, on hearing that I was a physician, asked me to do something "medical." So I kept him waiting. Then I sent him a bill.

— Clifford Kuhn, MD [246]

Most medical offices use computers only for billing purposes. This allows accountants to keep each record up to date, making sure that every patient quickly and efficiently receives the wrong bill. *— Mark DePaolis, MD* [109]

On a hospital charge after a very brief visit:
If I'd known his head in the door was worth $90, I would have made sure that it stayed there longer. *— Geraldine Merken* [215]

A fashionable surgeon, like a pelican, can be recognized by the size of his bill.

— J. Chalmers Da Costa, MD [102]

My doctor is a family physician. He treats my family and I support his.

— Phyllis Diller [269]

Physicians of the Utmost Fame
Were called at once, but when they came
They answered, as they took their Fees,
"There is no Cure for this Disease." *— Hilaire Belloc* [30]

"Tell me the truth doc," said Mr. Perot, "am I ever going to get well?"
   "Of course you are," replied the doctor. "You're going to get well if it costs every cent you have."

The receptionist called one of Dr. Cama's patients.
   "Mr. White, the check you gave us for your office visit came back."
   "Then we're even," White said. "So did my arthritis."

A patient went to the doctor for his annual checkup. After a thorough examination, the doctor said, "I've got some good news and some bad news."
   "What's the good news?" the patient said.
   "My son just got into Harvard Medical School."
   "And the bad news?"
   "You're paying for it."

Bobby Miller was a retired baseball player who was down on his luck and in need of an operation. He asked around and was referred to the most respected and expensive specialist in town.

"Doc, I've been told that I need this expensive operation," Miller explained.

"You're right," the doctor replied. "You do need the procedure, and it costs $20,000 to perform."

"C'mon, doc, times are tough. I didn't make the big bucks when I played ball so I can't afford that much."

"I'll tell you what I'll do," the doctor responded. "I used to be a big fan of yours, so I'll do it for $2,000 and one of your old uniforms."

"That's still to steep," the old ballplayer replied.

They haggled back and forth, and finally settled on $100 and a baseball cap the old timer wore in his last World Series.

As Miller got up to leave, the specialist said, "If you knew I was the most expensive doctor in town, why did you come to me?"

"Heck, doc," replied Miller. "where my health is concerned, money is no object."

A man who was having trouble with his sink called a plumber to his house. After the plumber checked the pipes, he leaned back and said, "I can fix the problem, but I want you to know that my fee is $200 per half hour."

"What!" said the startled man. "Why, I'm a neurosurgeon, and I only get $200 for a full hour."

"Hey, don't feel bad," the plumber said sympathetically. "When I was a neurosurgeon, I only made $200 an hour myself."

(See also Health Care Costs, Medical Practice)

~ BIOCHEMISTRY ~

(See Krebs Cycle)

~ BIOLOGIC CLOCK ~

I want to have children and I know my time is running out. I want to have them while my parents are still young enough to take care of them.   — *Rita Rudner* [322]

Sally: It's not the same for men. Charlie Chaplin had babies when he was 73.
Harry: Yes, but he was too old to pick them up.
— Nora Ephron, "When Harry Met Sally" [(123)]

(See also Motherhood)

~ BIRTH CONTROL ~

My husband and I found this great new method of birth control that really, really works. Every night before we go to bed, we spend an hour with our kids.
— Roseanne Barr [(135)]

I had a dream that all the victims of the pill came back. Boy, were they mad.
— Steven Wright [(135)]

The Jewish position on abortion is that a fetus is a fetus until it gets out of medical school.
— Anonymous [(268)]

A friend of mine confused her valium with her birth control pills—she had 14 kids but didn't give a damn.
— Joan Rivers [(217)]

There was a young lady from France
Who decided to take a big chance.
   She left her pills home
   And slept with Jerome;
Now all of her sisters are aunts.
— Anonymous [(217)]

I was involved in an extremely good example of oral contraception two weeks ago. I asked a girl to go to bed with me and she said "No."
— Woody Allen [(268)]

Contraceptives should be used on every conceivable occasion.
— Spike Milligan [(103)]

One of the best things people could do for their descendants would be to sharply limit the number of them.
— Olin Miller [(96)]

An elderly woman went to see her doctor. When the doctor asked why she was there, the woman replied, "I'd like to have some birth control pills."

"Mrs. Parker, you're 75 years old," the doctor said. "Why on earth would you want birth control pills?"

"Because they help me sleep better."

"How do they help you sleep better?" the doctor asked.

"I put them in my granddaughter's orange juice and I sleep like a baby."

What do you call people who use the rhythm method of birth control?
— Parents.

(See also Condoms, Health Care Books, Pregnancy, Sex Education)

~ BIRTHMARKS ~

I've got a friend who is a procrastinator—he didn't get a birthmark until he was eight years old.   — *Steven Wright* [194]

A motto for hypochondriacs:
There is no such thing as *just* a mole.   — *Fran Lebowitz* [190]

~ BLOOD & BLOOD DRAWING ~

The harder it is to find a patient's vein, the more likely it is that his CBC will clot.   — *Anonymous* [94]

Shumway's Law: Bleeding always stops. [201]

When drawing blood a good rule of thumb is that there should be at least as much blood in the tube as on your clothes.   — *Howard Bennett, MD* [48]

Referring to patients with poor venous access:
You can't get blood out of a turnip.   — *Anonymous* [94]

Drawing blood is a pain in the neck. First you have to tie a tourniquet around the patient's arm. Next you check out their veins until you find a nice juicy one and then ZAP, in goes the needle and blood's squirting all over the place. Why can't we fix people like they do on *Star Trek*? You know, wave that little thing over their body and say, "You're all better now. Come see me again if you develop any symptoms of Rigelian Flu." — *Molly Ryan, MD* [246]

Three vampires go into a bar for drinks. The first one orders blood. The second one orders blood. The third one orders plasma.

   The waitress calls out the order, "Two bloods and a blood lite."

(See also Lab Tests, Procedures)

~ BODILY FLUIDS ~

Bodily Fluids, n. Various substances that drip, ooze, or shoot out of patients— usually at the least opportune moment. — *Howard Bennett, MD* [46]

~ BODY ~

The body of a young woman is God's greatest achievement. . . Of course, He could have built it to last longer, but you can't have everything. — *Neil Simon* [288]

The human body is a beautiful thing, man, but beauty's only skin deep. Beneath the surface lurks a disgusting and frightening world of guts, gore, and glandular disorders. — *Bart Simpson* [149]

(See also Anatomy)

~ BRAIN ~

The brain is a wonderful organ; it starts the minute you wake up in the morning and does not stop until you get to the office. — *Robert Frost* [103]

He's very clever but sometimes his brains go to his head.   — *Margaret Asquith* [16]

Brain, n. What people are forced to use who don't have college degrees.
— *Anonymous* [71]

Science magazine came out with a report on the difference between men's and women's brains. Apparently women are controlled by a part of the brain called the cingulate gyrus and men are controlled by a part of the brain known as the penis.   — *Jay Leno* [135]

The brain uses less power than a 100-watt bulb. With lawyers, it's much less.
— *Anonymous* [135]

The chief function of your body is to carry your brain around.
— *Thomas Edison* [307]

The brain is an appendage of the genital glands.   — *Carl Jung* [71]

The human brain is a device to keep the ears from grating on one another.
— *Peter DeVries* [103]

My brain? It's my second favorite organ.   — *Woody Allen & Marshall Brickman* [5]

A doctor is hit by a car while crossing the street. He's taken to the closest emergency room and after a brief examination, the attending physician asks to speak with the doctor's wife. He explains, "Your husband has suffered severe brain damage, but thanks to new technology, we can do a brain transplant. Before we proceed, however, I think I should tell you how much it will cost. If you want him to have an internist's brain, it will cost $10 per pound. If you want a psychiatrist's brain, it will cost $25 per pound. And if you want a orthopedist's brain, it will cost $5,000 per pound."

"Good Heaven's," exclaimed the wife. "Why is it so expensive to get an orthopedist's brain?"

"Lady," said the doctor, "do you know how many orthopods we have to use to get a pound of brain?"

(See also Hypothalamus)

~ Breast Exams ~

I have a card with diagrams of how to do a breast exam hanging in my shower. Usually I leave the picture side facing the wall. However, one day the cleaning lady left it turned outward and my 7-year-old son Jake saw it and asked me what it was for. Without going into much detail, I told him it was there to remind me to do something every month and to show me how to do it. Jake replied: "Mama, I can't believe you don't know how to wash your boobs."

— *Peggy Johnson* [323]

During an examination on a flat-chested young woman, a medical student said, "Do you check yourself regularly for breast lumps?"

The woman replied, "I don't just check for breast lumps, I *pray* for breast lumps."

(See also Mammograms)

~ Breast Feeding ~

The *real* advantage of breast-feeding is that *only female persons can do it*. This means that male persons do not have to get up at the insane hours that babies like to get up. At first you may feel guilty about this, and you'll get up in the middle of the night to give the female person moral support. But after a while you'll get so good at morally supporting her that you'll be able to do it *without even waking up*.

— *Dave Barry* [24]

As a breastfeeding mother, you are basically meals on heels.

— *Kathy Lette* [194]

C

~ CADAVERS ~

When I die, I'm going to leave my body to science fiction.

— *Rodney Dangerfield* [135]

(See also Anatomy)

~ CAFFEINE ~

Caffeine is a powerful stimulant for the entire body, especially the part responsible for taking an unconscious, wrinkled mass of twisted bed sheets and matted hair and converting it into something resembling human form.

— *Mark DePaolis, MD* [109]

~ CANCER ~

It has recently been discovered that research causes cancer in rats.

— *Anonymous* [135]

On a report that suggested a possible health benefit from eating beef:
Saying that cheeseburgers help prevent cancer because they contain tiny amounts of an anticarcinogen makes as much sense as saying Attila the Hun was a nice guy because he once bought flowers for his mother.

— *Michael Jacobson, MD* [165]

Did you hear about the man who gradually gave up everything that doctors have linked to cancer?
• The first week, he cut out smoked fish and charcoal steaks.

- The second week, he cut out smoking.
- The third week, he cut out fatty foods.
- The fourth week, he cut out drinking.
- The fifth week, he cut out paper dolls.

A man goes to see his doctor for a checkup. After some tests, the doctor comes back with a serious look on his face. "I have some bad news and some really bad news," he says.

"Well, give me the really bad news first," the patient says.
"You have cancer and only six months to live."
"And the bad news?"
"You have Alzheimer's Disease."
"Thank God," the patient says. "I was afraid I had cancer."

~ CARDIAC ARREST ~

The first thing to do at a code is to check your own pulse.   — *Anonymous* [94]

On a man who used a toilet plunger to resuscitate his father during a heart attack:
We recommend that he take a basic CPR course, but it's hard to argue with success.   — *Keith Luri, MD* [62]

~ CARDIAC SURGERY ~

Heart surgeons don't have the world's smallest egos—when you ask them to name the world's three leading practitioners, they can never remember the names of the other two.   — *Sarah Paretsky* [237]

McDonald's "breakfast for under a dollar" actually costs much more than that. You have to factor in the cost of the coronary bypass surgery.
— *George Carlin* [135]

How many cardiac surgeons does it take to change a light bulb?
— One. He stands still while the world revolves around him.

A cardiac surgeon watched a mechanic as he removed engine parts from his car in order to get at the valves. After they introduced themselves, they began talking about their lines of work.

"You know doc," the mechanic said, "I think this type of work may be as complicated as the work you do."

"Perhaps," the surgeon replied, "but let's see you do it with the engine running."

After triple bypass surgery, Spencer was told he must stop smoking, drinking, and eating fatty foods.

"What about sex?" he asked his surgeon.

"Sex is fine," the doctor said, "but only with your wife. I don't want you to get too excited."

~ CARDIOLOGY ~

An aspirin a day keeps the cardiologist away.   — *Mark DePaolis, MD* [109]

I'm proud of being a workaholic. If it wasn't for people like me, cardiologists would loose half their business.   — *Ryan James, MD* [246]

Jack Sprat would eat no fat
His wife would eat no lean.
She was cath'd at 42,
And he choked on a bean.   — *Howard Bennett, MD* [45]

Bloopers & Malapropisms:
• The patient has chest pain if she lies on her left side for over a year.
• By the time the patient was admitted to the hospital her rapid heart had stopped and she was feeling much better.
• "My doctor put me on Lasix for *watery tension*." (water retention)
• Physical examination revealed a patent *foraminal valley*. (foramen ovale)
• The patient presented to the ER with chest pain, but *cereal* enzymes and an EKG were normal. (serial)
• Prior to admission, the patient was seen by a physician who at the time was in congestive heart failure.

- The patient is a 24-year-old white female with a history of *sinkable* episodes. (syncopal)
- The EKG revealed elevated P waves and a wandering *tape measure*. (pacemaker)
- The patient was 64 years old when he had his first myocardial *infraction*. (infarction)

A 92-year-old man went to see his doctor for a physical. A few days later, the doctor saw the man walking down the street with a beautiful young woman on his arm.

The following week, the old man went back to the doctor to get his test results. "You're really doing great aren't you?" the doctor said.

"Just following orders, doc," the old man replied. "Like you said, 'Get a hot mama and be cheerful'."

"I didn't say that," the doctor announced. "I said you had a heart murmur and told you to be careful."

(See also Arteries, Chest Pain, Cholesterol, EKG, Heart, High Blood Pressure)

~ CASE PRESENTATIONS ~

Managing a case presentation involves more than just reciting clinical information to your attending. It's an acquired skill, like salivating to the dinner bell, that is passed on from generation to generation.   — *Howard Bennett, MD* [32]

In the world of patients and places,
There's no room for those who botch cases.   — *Howard Bennett, MD* [32]

(See also Roundsmanship)

~ CASE REPORTS ~

Smith's Axiom on Publishing: One patient is a case report, two are a series. [135]

Breathes there a doc with soul so dead
Who never to himself has said,
"This is a case I should write up,
I'll do it tonight, before I sup!
Tomorrow, well-known I shall be,
They'll name a clinic after me."

— Naomi Bluestone, MD [56]

(See also Writing & Publishing)

~ CAT Scans ~

A CAT scan a day keeps the lawyers away.

— Howard Bennett, MD [40]

What do you give the hypochondriac who has everything?
— A CAT Scan.

(See also Radiology)

~ Cephalosporins ~

If we can't use them correctly, perhaps we can at least spell them correctly.

— Robert Ellis, Pharm.D. & Danny J. Lancaster, MD [120]

(See also Antibiotics)

~ Chest Pain ~

Chest Pain, n. The patient's trump card, his definitive demand for attention;
analogous to your mother's threat to tell your father, your father's threat to tell
your mother, or your wife's threat to tell everyone.

— George Thomas, MD & Lee Schreiner, MD [303]

My father was once rushed to the hospital from his hotel room with an apparent heart attack that, thank heavens, turned out to be an "acute gastric episode." That's the term hospitals use for five thousand dollars' worth of heartburn.

— *Christopher Buckley* [72]

(See also Cardiology, Heart)

~ CHICKEN SOUP ~

When I was younger, if any of us kids got sick, my mother would bring out the chicken soup. Of course, that didn't work for broken bones. For broken bones, she gave us boiled beef.

— *George Burns* [242]

(See also Common Cold)

~ CHIEF RESIDENT ~

Chief Residency, n. The first rung on the academic ladder in medicine. Responsibilities include making schedules, changing schedules, and arguing over schedules.

— *Howard Bennett, MD* [46]

How many chief residents does it take to change a light bulb?
— Just one, but five medical students follow him into the bathroom to watch him do it.

~ CHILDBIRTH ~

I think of birth as the search for a larger apartment.

— *Rita Mae Brown* [69]

Natural childbirth scares me. I think before you have natural childbirth you should find out how big the baby is. Three pounds—natural childbirth. Anything over three pounds—heroin.

— *Rita Rudner* [135]

Home delivery is for newspapers, not babies.

— Oscar Madison, "The Odd Couple" [(233)]

Amnesia: The condition that enables a woman who has gone through labor to have sex again.　　　　　　　　　　　　　　　　　　　*— Joyce Armor* [(13)]

On limiting the amount of time new mothers can stay in the hospital after delivery:
Naturally, these decisions are all made by men, who have no idea what it feels like to deliver a baby. Women know that any male who passed a seven-pound object through his own reproductive organs would be in intensive care for months, besides receiving years of therapy afterward.　　*— Mark DePaolis, MD* [(109)]

A friend asked her doctor if a woman should have children after thirty-five. I said, "Thirty-five children is enough for any woman."　　　*— Gracie Allen* [(76)]

People are giving birth underwater now. They say it's less traumatic for the baby because it's under water. But it's certainly more traumatic for the other people in the pool.　　　　　　　　　　　　　　　　　*— Elayne Boosler* [(67)]

President Clinton signed a bill that requires insurance companies to let mothers stay a minimum of 48 hours after their baby is born. To qualify, all the mother has to do is sign a form swearing that Bill Clinton isn't the father.　*— Jay Leno* [(135)]

I told my mother I was going to have natural childbirth. She said to me, "Linda, you've been taking drugs all your life. Why stop now?"　　*— Linda Maldonado* [(310)]

Having a baby is like taking your lower lip and forcing it over your head.

— Carol Burnett [(135)]

If men were the ones having babies, they would only do it once . . . maybe.

— Jan Henkelman [(246)]

Once my husband said to me, "I'm going to have some coffee. Do you want me to put some hot water on for you?" I thought that was the least he could do considering I was giving birth.　　　　　　　　　　　　　　*— Phyllis Diller* [(202)]

A telegram sent to a friend who had just given birth:
Congratulations! We all knew you had it in you. — *Dorothy Parker* [240]

A man calls the hospital and says, "You gotta help! My wife's going into labor."
   The nurse says, "Is this her first child?"
   "No," he says. "This is her husband."

A father asked his 4-year-old daughter what she would like for Christmas. Since her mom was 8 months pregnant, the girl said, "A baby sister."
   To everyone's delight, the mother came home on Christmas Eve with an 8 pound baby girl.
   Some time later, the father asked his daughter what she would like for Christmas the following year.
   "Well," the little girl said, "if it's not too uncomfortable for mom, I would like a pony."

(See also C-Sections, Pregnancy, Umbilical Cord)

~ CHILDREN ~

My kids will only eat three foods and two of them are macaroni and cheese.
   — *Rachel Ruina* [246]

Be nice to your children. After all, they are going to choose your nursing home.
   — *Steven Wright* [135]

The real menace in dealing with a 5-year-old is that in no time at all you begin to sound like a 5-year-old. — *Jean Kerr* [172]

Even when freshly washed and relieved of all obvious confections, children tend to be sticky. — *Fran Lebowitz* [195]

The main purpose of children's parties is to remind you that there are children worse than your own. — *Katharine Whitehorn* [194]

Familiarity breeds contempt—and children. — *Mark Twain* [19]

Ask your child what he wants for dinner only if he's buying.
— *Fran Lebowitz* [189]

The ideal age for children is when they're too old for baby-sitters, but too young to borrow the car. — *Robert Orben* [234]

Children today are tyrants. They contradict their parents, gobble their food, and tyrannize their teachers. — *Socrates* [268]

Any child can tell you that the sole purpose of a middle name is so he can tell when he's really in trouble. — *Dennis Fakes* [105]

Oh, what a tangled web do parents weave
When they think that their children are naïve. — *Ogden Nash (attrib.)* [217]

If you don't want your children to hear what you're saying, pretend you're talking to them. — *E. McKenzie* [196]

The quickest way for a parent to get a child's attention is to sit down and look comfortable. — *Lane Olinghouse* [217]

Nine-year-old Ryan came home from the playground with a torn shirt, a black eye, and a bloody nose. It was obvious he had been in a fight and lost. As his dad was patching him up, he asked his son what had happened.

"Well, dad," Ryan said, "I challenged Billy to a duel, and I gave him his choice of weapons."

"Uh-huh," said his father, "that seems fair."

"I know, but I never thought he'd choose his sister."

Two little boys were talking to each other on the playground when a little girl walked past.

One of the boys said, "When I stop hating girls, that's the one I'm going to stop hating first."

(See also Babies, Bedwetting, Food, Motherhood, Parenting, Sex Education, Thumb Sucking, Toilet Training, Youth)

~ CHILD SUPPORT ~

I was reading how a female spider will eat the male spider after mating. I guess female spiders know that life insurance is easier to collect than child support.
— *Janine DiTullio* [163]

(See also Divorce, Marriage)

~ CHIROPRACTORS ~

There are two times in a man's life when he shouldn't see a chiropractor—when he doesn't have back pain and when he does.   — *Ryan James, MD* [246]

How many chiropractors does it take to change a light bulb?
— Just one, but it takes twelve appointments.

(See also Acupuncture, Homeopathy)

~ CHOLESTEROL ~

Researchers have discovered that the traditional division between "good" and "bad" cholesterol is simplistic. There are actually six categories—appalling, pretty nasty, lard-belly, dry but full-flavored, perky, and basically okay once you get to know it.   — *Anonymous* [213]

I'm trying to eat better these days, so I buy all my groceries at Health Food stores. Just last week I ate some nitrite-free sausage. They're still 90% fat, but hey, it's *organic* fat.   — *Ryan James, MD* [246]

Cholesterol is a substance in the blood that causes you to eat salads.

— *Richard Carleton, MD* [83]

On a practical way to determine cholesterol levels:
Go to the trash can, open it up, and count the number of pizza boxes from Domino's. Now multiply by fifty.   — *Jay Leno* [135]

McDonald's "breakfast for under a dollar" actually costs much more than that. You have to factor in the cost of the coronary bypass surgery.

— *George Carlin* [135]

I love low fat. I'll buy anything that says *low fat*. They're not real specific though. They don't say lower than what. Lower than a great big old cup of fat?

— *Rita Rudner* [135]

The word cholesterol is taken from the Latin *chole* which means "bile," and *esterol*, meaning "substance that will clog all your arteries and cause your heart to wear out before your radial tires do."   — *Mark DePaolis, MD* [108]

Sing a song of lipids,
A stomach full of pie;
Four-and-twenty pastries
Sticking to your thighs.
When the pie is eaten
The chylomicrons sing;
Don't forget the Lipitor
Or you'll be wearing wings.   — *Howard Bennett, MD* [45]

A doctor finished examining one of his middle-aged patients and began to talk with him. "Mr. Robbins, I find very little wrong with you. You're in surprisingly good shape despite a borderline blood pressure and an elevated cholesterol count. However, if you want to stay healthy, my advice is that you stop eating all those eggs and start eating the cartons they come in."

(See also Cardiology, Food, Heart)

~ CHRONIC ~

Chronic, adj. Describing an entity that will not go away, despite the doctor's best efforts; sometimes a disease, often a patient.

— *George Thomas, MD & Lee Schreiner, MD* [303]

~ CIRCUMCISION ~

Circumcision, n. An elective surgical procedure that has persisted until modern times so adolescent males can shower at school in peace.

— *Howard Bennett, MD* [46]

A surgeon not known for precision
Decided on self-circumcision.
   One slip of the knife,
   "Oh dear!" cried his wife,
"Our love life will need some revision."

— *Anonymous* [316]

Never trust an obstetrician who says, "I'll just take a little off the top."

— *Ryan James, MD* [246]

Two 5-year-olds are sitting in a hospital waiting room. One leans over to the other and says, "What are you here for?"

"I have to be circumcised," the boy answers.

"Oh, man!" the first boy says. "I had that done five years ago, and I couldn't walk for twelve months."

Two men were standing at adjacent urinals when one said to the other, "I'll bet you were born in Newark, New Jersey."

"Why, that's right," said the second man.

"And I'll bet you were circumcised when you were three days old."

"Right again. But how'd you—"

"And I'll bet is was done by old Doc Myers."

"Why, yes, but how did you know?" asked the second man in amazement.

"Doc Myers always left too much foreskin," explained the first guy, "and you're peeing on my shoe."

A man was walking along the street in New York when he passed a jewelry shop. The man walked inside and said to the owner, "Could you repair my watch?"

The owner said, "I'm sorry, I don't repair watches."

"You don't repair watches? What do you do?"

"I'm a moyel."

"You're a moyel? Then why do you put all those watches in the window?" asked the man.

"Well, what would *you* put in the window?"

(See also Penis)

~ CLINICAL OBSERVATIONS ~

Pardee's Law: There is an inverse relationship between the uniqueness of an observation and the number of investigators who report it simultaneously. [201]

Rubinstein's Rule: It's hard to improve on the asymptomatic state. [202]

Fenagle's Laws on Information:
• The information you have is not what you want.
• The information you want is not what you need.
• The information you need is not what you can obtain. [201]

On common diagnoses occurring commonly:
When you hear hoofbeats think of horses, not zebras.   — *Anonymous* [94]

If it looks like a duck and sounds like a duck, it's probably a duck.
                                                              — *Anonymous* [94]

An elderly doctor decided it was time to turn over his medical practice to his son who had just finished his residency. Though well-versed in the latest medical advances, the son was unfamiliar with the nuances of small town practice. The old doctor took his son on some house calls to show him the ropes.

"One thing you always have to remember is that many times people won't tell you what you need to know to make a diagnosis. The first rule is that you must always be observant. For instance, Mrs. Carson is overweight, but her problem isn't glandular—she stuffs herself with candy bars. I saw dozens of empty wrappers in her garbage when I visited her the other day. And Mr. Wade complains that he has no energy, but that's because he drinks his dinner—I had to climb over a pile of Scotch bottles to get into his house last week. So remember, be observant."

At their first stop, the older doctor knocked on the door. When there was no response, the two of them entered and went upstairs to investigate. They found a beautiful women in bed with the sheets pulled up to her chin. The woman told them about her problem—she was having anxiety attacks. The younger doctor noticed beads of sweat on her forehead. He decided to take her temperature, but fumbled with the thermometer and it fell on the floor. He bent over to pick it up and went on with his examination.

When he finished the examination, he made his diagnosis. "I think you're getting too involved in politics," he said. "If you stop concentrating so much on that, I guarantee your attacks will subside." The woman sat up in bed and nervously thanked him.

As the doctors got back to their car, the older one said, "Why on earth did you give her that advice?"

"Just following your rule of simple observation, dad. When I bent over to pick up the thermometer, I noticed the mayor under the bed."

(See also Diagnosis, Experience)

~ CLINICAL PRACTICE GUIDELINES ~

Clinical Practice Guidelines, n. Cliff's Notes for doctors.
— *Howard Bennett, MD* [46]

~ CLONING ~

With cloning, everyone will be able to have all the children they want, allowing humans to procreate randomly without conscious thought or even dating.
— *Mark DePaolis, MD* [108]

If you clone one of your kids, is the new child more likely to listen to your advice than the original?
— *Ludwig Lettau, MD* [246]

There are two guys who are trying to clone human genes into cows so you'd get cows that would give human milk. Or maybe you'd get girls with four really big breasts . . . I'm sure they think, "Either way, big improvement."

— Cathryn Michon [(67)]

I saw the sequel to the movie *Clones*, and you know what? It was the same movie. *— Jim Samuels* [(89)]

(See also Genetics)

~ CLUB FOOT ~

I was born with a club foot. Had to wear orthopedic shoes with a brace on one side, so I used to walk with a limp. Thank God I lived in the ghetto, because the people who didn't know me thought I was cool—"Hey man, check out this brother's walk. He must be in a gang or something." *— Damon Wayans* [(135)]

~ CO-DEPENDENT ~

I'm not co-dependent myself, but aren't they great to have around?

— Betsy Salkind [(135)]

~ COLDS ~

(See Common Cold)

~ COLON ~

Colon, n. The light at the end of the tunnel; an organ of splendid promise, but disappointing performance. *— George Thomas, MD & Lee Schreiner, MD* [(303)]

~ COLONOSCOPY ~

Reality is what happens when you get your first colonoscopy.   — *Anonymous* [135]

You never realize how long a minute is until you've had a colonoscopy.
                                          — *Howard Bennett, MD* [48]

On the link between a sedentary lifestyle and colon cancer:
Colonoscopy is very sedentary work. Maybe we should do five pushups after
each procedure?   — *Moshe Shike, MD* [285]

A colonoscopy is nature's way of telling you to eat a low fat diet.
                                          — *Ryan James, MD* [246]

(See also Endoscopy, Gastrointestinal Tract, Proctology)

~ COMMITTEES ~

Wangensteen's Rule: Never turn down a hospital committee appointment and,
once appointed, never go. [216]

A committee is a group of individuals who singly can do nothing but who can
together agree that nothing can be done.   — *Fred Allen* [75]

To get something done a committee should consist of no more than three men,
two of whom are absent.   — *Robert Copeland* [217]

Nothing is impossible until it is sent to a committee.   — *J. H. Boren* [59]

(See also Academia, Meetings)

~ Common Cold ~

A remedy for the common cold:
Go to bed. Put a hat on the bedpost. Drink whiskey until you see two hats.
— *William Osler (attrib.)* [236]

If you catch a cold and don't attend to it, it will last fourteen days. But if you see a doctor and take the medicine he prescribes, you can get rid of it in two weeks.
— *Gracie Allen* [104]

Doctors still don't know what to do about colds. So now when I get one, I sit in a draft till it develops into something they can cure.
— *Rita Rudner* [135]

For my birthday I got a humidifier and a dehumidifier. I put them in the same room and let them fight it out.
— *Steven Wright* [135]

It's bad enough to have a cold,
And yet one may endure it,
If every friend would not proceed
To tell us how to cure it.
— *Francis Leo Golden, MD* [141]

The actress Billie Burke was dining in a restaurant where, at the next table, a man was obviously suffering from a bad cold. "I can see you're very uncomfortable," she volunteered. "So I'll tell you what to do for it—drink lots of orange juice and take lots of aspirin. When you go to bed, cover yourself with as many blankets as you can find. Sweat the cold out. Believe me, I know what I'm talking about. I am Billie Burke of Hollywood." The man smiled and introduced himself in return: "Thank you. I am Dr. Mayo of the Mayo Clinic." [320]

This woman sneezed like 300 times. She said, "There must be something in the air." I said, "Yeah, your germs."
— *Linda Herskovic* [62]

On treating the common cold:
A good gulp of whiskey at bedtime—it's not very scientific, but it helps.
— *Alexander Fleming* [103]

(See also Chicken Soup, Cough)

~ COMPLIANCE ~

The only way a patient will get better on a QID medication is if he didn't need it in the first place.
— *Molly Ryan, MD* [246]

A gray-haired woman went to the doctor complaining of swollen ankles. The doctor gave her anti-swelling pills and instructed her to take one every other day.
"I'm sorry, Doctor," said the lady. "I'm not sure I understand the treatment."
"It's very simple," said the doctor. "Take one pill today, skip tomorrow, take one pill the next day, skip the day after that, and continue that way until the prescription is finished. Then come back and see me."
A few weeks later, the woman returned, and her ankles looked completely normal. The doctor was pleased. "It looks like it worked. I think you can stop the medication."
"Oh, good," the woman said. "I didn't mind the pills, but the skipping was killing me."

(See also Advice)

~ COMPLICATIONS ~

No matter what you do, the number of complications will double if a patient or his spouse is either a physician or a nurse.
— *Anonymous* [94]

In the event of a complication, always blame the PMD.
— *Anonymous* [94]

My wife and I had all the complications you'd expect at a doctor's delivery—the epidural didn't work, they had to use forceps, and my mother-in-law stayed for three weeks.
— *Ryan James, MD* [246]

~ Compulsive Behavior ~

(See Obsessive-Compulsive Behavior)

~ Computers ~

To err is human, but to really screw things up requires a computer.

— *Anonymous* [283]

Never let a computer know you're in a hurry.   — *Anonymous* [75]

My computer caught a health care virus. It goes through your system for hours, finds nothing wrong, and sends you a bill for $2,500.   — *Anonymous* [135]

Most medical offices use computers only for billing purposes. This allows accountants to keep each record up to date, making sure that every patient quickly and efficiently receives the wrong bill.   — *Mark DePaolis, MD* [109]

~ Condoms ~

One of my friends found a condom on the verandah. When he questioned his teenage son about it, the kid replied, "What's a verandah?"   — *Lewis Grizzard* [148]

Condoms aren't completely safe. A friend of mine was wearing one and got hit by a bus.   — *Bob Rubin* [75]

Read the condom boxes, they're pretty funny. Trojans say, "New Shape." I didn't know this was necessary. Must have been that Chernobyl incident.

— *Elayne Boosler* [135]

National Condom Week is coming soon. Hey, there's a parade you won't want to miss.   — *Jay Leno* [135]

Bad luck is meeting your date's father and realizing he's the pharmacist you bought condoms from that afternoon.
— *Lewis Grizzard* [148]

An attractive young woman got caught in a sudden rainstorm. By the time she got under cover, she was drenched and needed a cigarette. A friend standing nearby reached into her pocket and pulled out a small rubber thing, unrolled it, and took out a perfectly dry cigarette. It was in a condom.

The woman said, "That's a great idea. I'll have to try it."

So the next day she went to a drugstore and said, "A package of condoms, please."

"What kind?" asked the pharmacist.

"I'm not sure," the woman said. "I guess it should be big enough for a Camel."

(See also Birth Control, Sex Education)

~ CONFERENCES ~

(See Continuing Medical Education)

~ CONJUNCTIVITIS ~

The best way to treat conjunctivitis in a small child is to put the drops in your dog's eyes and pray for a miracle.
— *Larry Bauer, MD* [246]

~ CONSTIPATION ~

Said the doc to the man constipated,
"Don't you think this complaint could have waited?
It's five after three,
So take it from me,
What you need is your head lubricated."
— *Howard Bennett, MD* [41]

Constipation means going to the bathroom less frequently than your mother.
— *Anonymous* [94]

There is no such thing as refractory constipation. There is only not enough Milk of Magnesia.
                                                                    — *Anonymous* [135]

According to statistics, a man eats a prune every 20 seconds. I don't know who this fellow is, but I know where to find him.
                                                                    — *Anonymous* [134]

An irregular patient named Krauss
Had the habit of calling my house.
  Said my wife with a grin,
  "Put the enema in,
And just wait for a call from my spouse."   — *Rick Stevens, MD* [246]

Old Mrs. Shaw went to her doctor complaining of constipation.
  "Do you do anything about it?" asked the doctor.
  "Of course I do. I sit on the toilet for two hours every day."
  "No, I don't mean that. I mean do you take anything?"
  "Of course," said the woman, "I take my knitting."

~ Continuing Medical Education ~

Medical conferences are always held at nice locations—this is based on the educational principle that to learn anything important, you must be able to swim or ski afterwards.
                                                                    — *Mark DePaolis, MD* [107]

Oh, we're off to a medical meeting
Where there's never a problem with seating,
  Except at the bar,
  Where friends from afar,
Are exchanging their annual greeting.   — *David Goldblatt, MD* [140]

I love a finished speaker,
I really, really do.
I don't mean one who's polished.
I just mean one who's through.   — *Richard Armour, Ph.D.* [269]

(See also Medical Literature)

~ CORONER ~

Dr. Frasier Crane (to a caller): And while I agree that washing his hands twenty to thirty times a day would be considered obsessive-compulsive behavior, bear in mind that your husband *is* a coroner.   — *"Frasier"* [131]

The easiest job in the world has to be a coroner. What's the worst thing that can happen? If everything went wrong, maybe you'd get a pulse.
                                                                         — *Dennis Miller* [139]

(See also Pathology)

~ COUGH ~

People with chronic coughs never seem to go to the doctor—they go to banquets, concerts, and church.   — *Anonymous* [135]

Frogs make excellent cough suppressants. To get rid of a cough put a live frog in your mouth, then release it. Repeat three times. The cough should disappear. Maybe.   — *Bart Simpson* [149]

The best way to stop a cough is to make an appointment to see the doctor.
                                                                         — *Larry Bauer, MD* [246]

He received from some thoughtful relations,
A spittoon with superb decorations.
   When asked was he pleased,
   He grimaced and wheezed,
"It's beyond all my expectorations."   — *Anonymous* [85]

A cough is something that you yourself can't help, but everybody else does on purpose just to torment you.   — *Ogden Nash* [229]

(See also Common Cold)

~ CPR ~

(See Cardiac Arrest)

~ C-SECTIONS ~

I recently attended a C-section and the father was in there videotaping the entire procedure. I'm thinking, who is he going to show *this* to? Guests that won't leave?
— Stu Silverstein, MD [246]

I was born by C-section. That was the last time I had my mother's complete attention.
— Richard Jeni [96]

When the doctor asked me if I wanted a bikini cut for my C-section, I said, "No! A bikini and a wine cooler is why I'm laying here now."
— Kim Tavares [67]

(See also Childbirth)

𝒟

~ DEATH ~

Death, n. The final effort of the patient to embarrass his physician publicly.
— *George Thomas, MD & Lee Schreiner, MD* [(303)]

When a patient is at death's door, it is the doctor's job to pull him through.
— *Anonymous* [(94)]

One can survive anything nowadays except death.
— *Oscar Wilde* [(206)]

According to an ad hoc committee at Harvard Medical school, a person is dead when the following criteria are met:
• His fingernails stop growing.
• He won't smile even when tickled.
• Blue Cross stops his payments.
• He graduates from Yale.
— *Anthony Shaw, MD* [(278)]

I'm not afraid of death. I just don't want to be there when it happens.
— *Woody Allen* [(7)]

I get up each morning and dust off my wits,
Then pick up the paper and read the "obits."
If my name isn't there, then I know I'm not dead.
I eat a good breakfast and go back to bed.
— *Anonymous* [(184)]

Death, n. (an epidemiologist's definition): The ultimate state of the final common pathway that emerges subsequent to a terminal morbid event culminating in the eventual biocessation of animate bioprocesses.
— *Thomas B. Newman, MD & Warren S. Browner, MD* [(231)]

Here I am dying of a hundred good symptoms.
— *Alexander Pope* [(298)]

Martin Levine passed away at age 75. Mr. Levine owned a chain of movie theaters here in New York. The funeral will be held on Thursday at 2:15, 4:20, 6:30, 8:40, and 10:50. — *David Letterman* [135]

The key, I think, is to not think of death as an end, but to think of it more as a very effective way to cut down on your expenses. — *Woody Allen* [6]

During his last illness, W.C. Fields was confined to a hospital bed. When a visitor saw him reading the Bible, Fields said, "Just looking for loopholes." [320]

In this world nothing is certain, except death and taxes. — *Benjamin Franklin* [283]

For three days after death, hair and fingernails continue to grow, but phone calls taper off. — *Johnny Carson* [217]

I am ready to meet my Maker. Whether my Maker is prepared for the ordeal of meeting me is another matter. — *Winston Churchill* [103]

It's a funny world—a man's lucky if he can get out alive. — *W. C. Fields* [217]

Death is nature's way of telling you to slow down. — *Dick Sharples* [249]

When I die, I want to go peacefully like my grandfather did, in his sleep. Not screaming, like the passengers in his car. — *Michael Jeffreys* [89]

Mr. Thomas went to the doctor and found out that he only had ten hours to live. Rushing home, he told his wife the bad news.

"Honey," she said. "Let's go to bed. I'm going to make this the most memorable ten hours of your life."

After they got undressed, the woman did everything her husband ever wanted a woman to do. When they finished, Mr. Thomas asked her to do it again. She knew it would take a lot of strength and determination, but she did as he asked.

When they finished, it was 3 o'clock in the morning and the woman was completely spent. As she lay on her back, Mr. Thomas asked her to do it one more time. She looked him straight in the eye and said, "Sure, what do you care? You don't have to get up in the morning."

As an elderly patient neared his end, his relatives came by to pay their final respects. But as is often the case, they started telling him how much better he looked. "Your color's better," one of them said. "The doctor says your heart sounds more regular," another added. "And you seem to be breathing easier," a third told him.

"That's nice," the old man replied. "It's reassuring to know that I'm going to die in such good shape."

Two old docs in their eighties had been playing golf together for years. One day they got to talking about life after death.

"Do you think there's golf in heaven?" one of them asked.

"I sure hope so," the other replied. "I'll tell you what. Let's make a pact. Whoever dies first will come back and tell the other."

Sure enough, about three weeks later the first fellow died. Shortly thereafter, as his friend lay in bed, he heard a voice.

"John? Is that you?"

"Yes, it's me. And I've come back to tell you about heaven."

"So tell me, do they have golf up there?"

"Well, I've got good news and bad news. The good news is yes, there is golf in heaven. The fairways are all lush and green, and everybody shoots par or better."

"So what's the bad news?"

"The bad news is that you've got a tee time next Wednesday."

A son was sitting at the bedside of his elderly father, who was dying. "Where do you want to be buried," asked the son, "Forest Lawn or New York City?"

The old man got up on his elbow and said, "Oh, I don't know son. Why don't you just surprise me?"

A man on a business trip calls his wife to see how things are at home. At the end of the conversation, he asks about the family cat.

"He's dead," the wife answers abruptly.

The man is devastated. "You know how much Oliver meant to me," he sobs into the phone. "Couldn't you be a little more sensitive? Why didn't you break the news gently? You could have said, 'Well, honey, Oliver got out of the house the other day and he climbed up on the roof. The fire department tried, but they couldn't get him down and he died of exposure or starvation.' You're an internist for heaven's sake. Is that how you talk to your patients?"

The wife apologizes and tells her husband she'll try to do better next time.

After he calms down, the husband says, "By the way, how's mom?"

The wife pauses for a moment, then says, "Mom's on the roof."

An intern was taking a history on a new patient in the clinic. "You seem to be in excellent health, Mrs. Malloy. Could you tell me what your parents died of?"

"I can't remember," the patient answered. "But I'm sure it was nothing serious."

(See also Last Words, Old Age)

~ DEPRESSION ~

The price of Prozac went up 50% last year. When they asked Prozac users how they felt about this they said, "Whatever . . ."   — *Conan O'Brien* [135]

There is evidence that Prozac improves all functions of the brain, even the ones that keep track of car keys.   — *Mark DePaolis, MD* [108]

I had to get rid of my therapist; she wasted a lot of time talking. So I said, "Excuse me, but can we go directly to the medication?"   — *Maura Kennedy* [67]

I take Prozac, therefore I am.   — *Anonymous* [135]

My friends said to me, "Margaret, you're down. Take the Prozac. Take the Zoloft. Take the Paxil." They're all on it. Now I feel better. . . I guess it was them.   — *Margaret Smith* [67]

How many psychopharmacologists does it take to change a light bulb?
— None. Most would diagnose depression and prescribe Zoloft instead.

~ DERMATOLOGY ~

A dermatologist is someone who tells you in Latin what you just told him in English.   — *Anonymous* [94]

Dermatologists always sleep through the night.   — *Anonymous* [94]

Dermatology is the perfect specialty—patients never get well, they never die, and they never call at night.
— *Wayman R. Spence, MD* [291]

Skin doesn't need a doctor. Wash it. Dry it. Move on!
— *George Castanza, "Seinfeld"* [276]

Urticaria, n. Indicative of a desire to be manually transported by a third person; as, "The only reason that kid is screaming at her mother is that she wants urticaria."
— *H. S. Grannatt* [145]

Bloopers & Malapropisms:
• Skin: Somewhat pale but present.
• A 16-year-old male presented with a rash in his *generals*. (genitals)
• Past medical history is positive for eczema and *contract* dermatitis. (contact)
• The patient is a 28-year-old who presented with a pyogenic *granola*. (granuloma)
• Two days after starting an antibiotic, the patient presented with an *expensive* rash. (extensive)
• Examination of the abdomen revealed a large *pediculus*. (panniculus)
• The plantar wart was *defecated*. (desiccated)
• The patient, who is allergic to cats, presented with generalized *purritis*. (pruritus)
• The patient's condition is consistent with Letterer-*Seaweed* disease. (Siwe)
• Mr. Watson is a 46-year-old man whose chief complaint is a rash on his *grand penis*. (glans)
• While speaking to the triage nurse about a genital rash, the patient said, "I just want you to know that I'm married and we're *monotonous*." (monogamous)

Rules of Dermatology:
• If it's wet, dry it.
• If it's dry, wet it.
• If it's neither wet nor dry, use steroids.
• If steroids don't work, do a biopsy.
— *Anonymous* [94]

Updated Rules of Dermatology:
• If it's wet, dry it.
• If it's dry, wet it.
• But whatever you do, don't touch it.
— *Anonymous* [94]

Dermatology Definitions:
• Annular: Occurring once a year.
• Bullae: A tough guy.
• Cauterize: What the intern did before he winked at his date.
• Currette: A partial recovery.
• Duct: Avoided being hit.
• Fester: Quicker.
• Friable: Can be cooked.
• Kerion: What you take with you during a flight.

A man says to his dermatologist, "How much will it cost to get this mole removed?"
    "About $300."
    "Three hundred dollars for just a few minutes work?"
    The dermatologist says, "I can remove it very slowly if you like."

How many dermatologists does it take to change a light bulb?
— Just one, but he won't do it after 5PM or on weekends.

What three things can the average person do in a minute and a half?
— Drink a soda, eat a brownie, and have an appointment with a dermatologist.

What's the difference between an itch and a rash?
— About $150.

(See also Baldness, Birthmarks, Itching, Lyme Disease, Varicose Veins)

~ DIAGNOSIS ~

A well person is a patient who has not been completely worked up.
— J. Freymann, MD [132]

The more often you put your finger (or an instrument) in an orifice, the less often you will put your foot in your mouth.   — Rip Pfeiffer, MD [248]

Rubinstein's Observation:
It takes a healthy person to survive a full medical workup. [203]

When in doubt, write illegibly. — *Howard Bennett, MD* [40]

Doctors hate to be wrong. My internist made the wrong diagnosis once. I said, "Did you miss this one Jim?" He shook his head and told me I had the wrong symptoms. — *Larry Bauer MD* [246]

Clinical Practice Guidelines, n. Cliff's Notes for doctors. — *Howard Bennett, MD* [46]

Notice in a doctor's waiting room:
To avoid delay, please have all of your symptoms ready. — *Anonymous* [94]

Three doctors were on their way to a conference when their car got a flat. They all got out of the car and inspected the tire. The first doctor said, "I think it's flat."

The second doctor examined it closely and said, "It sure looks flat."

The third doctor felt the tire and said, "It feels like a flat."

All three nodded their heads and said, "Let's run some tests."

A pair of retired internists were having lunch in Central Park when a man walked towards them. The man was bent at the waist, his feet were pointing inward, and his arms were held close to his chest.

"So, Abe," one of the doctors said. "You still think you've got what it takes to diagnose patients?"

"Sure, I do. You want me to tell you what that man has? It's obvious he's suffering from rheumatoid arthritis."

"I disagree," the other doctor said. "Look at his gait. It's obvious that he recently had a stroke."

Before they could argue the merits of their observations, the man stopped in front of them and said, "Excuse me gentlemen, could you please tell me where the bathrooms are around here?"

(See also Bodily Fluids, Clinical Observations, Experience, Lab Tests, Physical Examination, Procedures, Second Opinions, Symptoms)

~ DIAPERS ~

A bit of talcum
Is always walcum.
— *Ogden Nash* [217]

A soiled baby, with a neglected nose, cannot be conscientiously regarded as a thing of beauty.
— *Mark Twain* [268]

Any mother with half a skull knows that when Daddy's little boy becomes Mommy's little boy, the kid is so wet he's treading water.
— *Erma Bombeck* [243]

In the world of babies and diapers,
There's no hope for those who are wipers.
— *Howard Bennett, MD* [32]

(See also Babies)

~ DIAPHRAGM ~

The diaphragm is a muscular partition that separates disorders of the chest from disorders of the bowels.
— *Ambrose Bierce* [51]

~ DIARRHEA ~

The quickest way to cure diarrhea is to request a stool sample.
— *Anonymous* [94]

Diarrhea and constipation can be loosely defined as going to the bathroom more or less frequently than your mother.
— *Anonymous* [94]

A new report from the government says that raw eggs may have salmonella and can be unsafe. In fact, the latest theory says it wasn't the fall that killed Humpty Dumpty—he was dead before he hit the ground.
— *Jay Leno* [135]

The good thing about food poisoning is that Americans can experience exotic infections without the expense and inconvenience of having to travel to another country. — *Ludwig Lettau, MD* [246]

Little Jack Horner
Sat in the corner,
Eating an undercooked pie;
He got salmonella,
Was a pretty sick fella,
And said, "What a dumb cluck am I!" — *Howard Bennett, MD* [45]

~ DIETING ~

I went on a diet. Had to go on two diets at the same time 'cause one wasn't giving me enough food. — *Barry Marter* [135]

The older you get, the harder it is to lose weight because your body has made friends with your fat. — *Lynne Alpern & Esther Blumenfeld* [195]

I've been on a diet for two weeks and all I've lost is two weeks. — *Totie Fields* [134]

Before going on a diet you should consult your doctor, or at least send him some money. — *Dave Barry* [24]

If you are the sort of person who always thinks she needs to go on a diet, realize this: everything will always make you fat for the rest of your life. This is especially true if you live with someone who never gains weight. It is due to a little-known phenomenon called *Secondary Weight Gain.* — *Merrill Markoe* [198]

The second day of a diet is always easier than the first. By the second day, you're off of it. — *Jackie Gleason* [135]

The most difficult part of a diet isn't watching what you eat. It's watching what other people eat. — *Anonymous* [218]

Now I sit me down to eat,
I pray the Lord my weight to keep,
If I should reach for cake or bread,
Please guide my hand to fish instead. — *Anonymous* [166]

I've got a doctor's appointment on Monday. I'm not sick or anything. It's just that I lost some weight, and I want someone to see me naked.

— *Tracy Smith* [67]

There are four basic food groups: salad, hors d'oeuvres, pasta, and diet drinks.

— *Merrill Markoe* [198]

A good reducing exercise consists of placing both hands against the table edge and pushing back. — *Anonymous* [125]

Eat, drink, and be merry, for tomorrow we may diet. — *Harry Kurnitz* [268]

I feel about dieting the way I feel about airplanes. It seems to me they are wonderful things for other people to go on. — *Jean Kerr* [217]

Successful dieting is a triumph of mind over platter. — *Anonymous* [219]

Never eat anything at one sitting that you cannot lift. — *Miss Piggy* [217]

Nothing in the world arouses more false hope than the first four hours of a diet.

— *Anonymous* [186]

If you wish to grow thinner, diminish your dinner. — *H. S. Leigh* [249]

Rules of Dieting:
• If no one sees you eat it, it has no calories.
• If you drink a diet soda with a candy bar, they cancel each other out.
• When eating with someone else, calories don't count if you both eat the same thing.
• Food used for medicinal purposes never counts, such as hot chocolate, brownies, and Sara Lee cheesecake. [135]

The doctor finished his examination as his patient struggled to pull his pants over his forty-six inch waist. "Mr. Benson, you've really put on weight since your last exam," the doctor said. "I'm putting you on a special low-fat, low-calorie diet. Six months from now, I want to see two thirds of you back in my office."

A panhandler walked up to a woman who was about to go into a coffee shop and said, "Lady, I haven't eaten in a week."

"Wow!" exclaimed the woman. "I wish I had your will power."

There was a thin maiden named Lena
Who purchased a new vacuum cleaner.
   But she got in the way
   Of its suction one day
And since then, no one has seen her.   *— Francis Leo Golden, MD* [141]

(See also Food, Obesity)

~ DIPLOMA ~

A doctor is the happiest twice in his life—the day he hangs his diploma up and the day he takes it down.   *— Howard Bennett, MD* [40]

A diploma is a remembrance of things passed.   *— Honey Greer* [168]

Your diploma only starts you in practice; it's your diplomacy that keeps you there.   *— Philip A. Kilbourne, MD* [176]

(See also Education)

~ DISABILITIES ~

(See Handicaps)

~ Disease ~

Disease, n. Nature's endowment to medical schools. — *Ambrose Bierce* [51]

During an episode of the sitcom, "Maude," the characters were hosting a telethon, but they had yet to come up with a disease to sponsor. At one point, someone said, "You can't take money from people without knowing what the disease is." Maude answered, "Why not, doctors do it all the time." [204]

My diseases are an asthma and a dropsy and, what is less curable, seventy-five.
— *Samuel Johnson* [219]

The Art of Medicine consists of amusing the patient while nature cures the disease. — *Voltaire* [268]

(See also Complications, Illness, Symptoms)

~ Divorce ~

Relationships don't last anymore. When I meet a guy, the first question I ask myself is, "Is this the man I want my children to spend their weekends with?"
— *Rita Rudner* [135]

Alimony is always having to say you're sorry. — *Philip J. Simborg* [75]

Divorce dates from just about the same time as marriage. I think marriage is a few weeks older. — *Voltaire* [268]

I heard that dysfunctional family guru John Bradshaw is going through a divorce. I suppose the big question is, who will get custody of his inner child?
— *Stu Silverstein, MD* [246]

There is so little difference between husbands, you might as well keep the first.
— *Adela Rogers St. Johns* [311]

Our parents got divorced when we were kids and it was kind of cool. We got to go to divorce court with them. It was like a game show. My mom won the house and car. We were all excited. My dad got some luggage.   — *Tom Arnold* [163]

A couple in their nineties filed for divorce. A friend of the family asked the woman why, after 70 years of marriage, they decided to split up.

"Our marriage had been on the rocks for quite some time," the woman answered, "but we wanted to wait until the children died."

(See also Child Support, Marriage)

~ DOCTOR-PATIENT COMMUNICATION ~

Doctors are not allowed to tell you directly what is wrong—this would be a breach of ethics—so you have to listen closely to their muttering and interpret it. Here are the standard doctor mutters, translated into laymen's terms:
• *Uh-huh:* This means, "Oh my God."
• *Ummm:* This means, "Good Lord."
• *Ah hah:* This means, "I vaguely remember seeing a case like this in medical school, but it hadn't advanced nearly this far."   — *Dave Barry* [24]

It's impossible to get doctors on the phone. I've tried. Every so often I call my own office just to see, and I can't get me. The best I can do is to leave a message, and even then it takes me two or three days to get back to myself.
— *Mark DePaolis, MD* [110]

"Hello," the caller said to the nurse. "You have a patient named Jonathan Ross on your floor. Can you tell me how he's doing?"

"He's doing fine," the nurse said. "The doctor removed his stitches this morning and expects he'll be discharged in a day or two."

"Thanks," said the caller.

"Would you like to tell Mr. Ross that you called?"

"This is Mr. Ross," the caller said. "My doctor doesn't stay in the room long enough to tell me anything."

"You seem to be recovering nicely," the doctor said. "These x-rays show some damage to the bone, but I wouldn't worry about it."

The patient said, "If your bones were damaged, I wouldn't worry about it either."

(See also Bedside Manner, Ethics)

~ DOCTORS ~

Dammit, Jim, I'm a doctor, not a bricklayer!
— *Leonard "Bones" McCoy, MD, "Star Trek"* [294]

Doctors must go to school for years and years, often with little sleep and with great sacrifice to their first wives. — *Roy Blount Jr* [29]

If you grow up Jewish in New York, you basically have three career choices— You can become a doctor, a lawyer, or a doctor. — *Stu Silverstein, MD* [246]

Women go after doctors like men go after models. They want someone with knowledge of the body. We just want the body. — *Jerry Seinfeld, "Seinfeld"* [276]

Remember, half the doctors in the country graduated in the bottom half of their class. — *Al McGuire* [197]

A physician who treats himself has a fool for a patient. — *William Osler, MD* [298]

It is amazing what little harm doctors do when one considers all the opportunities they have. — *Mark Twain* [135]

My doctor is nice; every time I see him I'm ashamed of what I think about doctors in general. — *Mignon McLaughlin* [247]

According to a recent survey, 50% of physicians said they would rather play a doctor on TV than be one in real life. — *Howard Bennett, MD* [48]

Never go to a doctor whose office plants have died. — *Erma Bombeck* [29]

I used to play doctor with this little girl in my neighborhood all the time. One time we got caught. Luckily, it was a Wednesday and we were just playing golf.

— *Brian Kiley* [163]

It's a good idea to "shop around" before you settle on a doctor. Ask about the condition of his Mercedes. Ask about the competence of his mechanic. Don't be shy! After all, you're paying for it. — *Dave Barry* [322]

Doctors should never talk to patients about anything but medicine. When doctors talk politics, economics or sports, they reveal themselves to be ordinary mortals—you know, idiots like the rest of us. — *Andy Rooney* [62]

Our doctor would never really operate unless it was necessary. He was just that way. If he didn't need the money, he wouldn't lay a hand on you. — *Herb Shriner* [29]

Two society women had lunch at a Palm Springs hotel.

"You ought to try my doctor," Mrs. Green said to her friend. "He's really marvelous."

"Why should I see your doctor?" Mrs. Van Brackle said. "There's nothing wrong with me."

"Well," replied Mrs. Green, "my doctor's wonderful. He'll find something."

A doctor dies and goes to heaven, where he finds a long line at St. Peter's gate. As is his custom, the doctor rushes to the front, but St. Peter tells him to go wait in line like everyone else. Muttering and looking at his watch, the doctor stands at the end of the line.

Moments later, a white-haired man carrying a stethoscope and black bag rushes to the front of the line, waves to St. Peter, and is immediately admitted through the pearly gates.

"Hey!" the doctor says angrily. "How come you let him through without waiting?"

"Oh," says St. Peter, "that's God. Sometimes he likes to play doctor."

Old Doc Wellner passed away, and a group of his friends decided to collect some money to give him a nice funeral. Their collection was a little short, so they called on an eccentric rich man who lived in town.

"What do you want from me?" the old man snarled.

"Fifty dollars, to bury Doc Wellner," suggested the leader.

The old gentleman took out his checkbook and said, "Here's $300. Bury six of them."

A doctor is stranded on a desert island for ten years. One day, he sees a speck on the horizon. He thinks to himself, "Could it be a ship?" The speck gets a little closer and he thinks, "It's not a boat." The speck gets even closer and he thinks, "It's not a raft." Then, out of the water comes a beautiful redhead, wearing a wetsuit and scuba gear. She comes up to the physician and says, "How long has it been since you've had a fine cigar?"

"Ten years," he replies.

She unzips a waterproof pocket on her left sleeve and pulls out a nice Cuban cigar. He lights it, takes a long drag and says, "Man, is that good."

Then she asks, "How long has it been since you've had a glass of fine brandy?"

"Ten years," he replies.

She unzips a pocket on her right sleeve and pulls out a flask filled with 100-year-old brandy. He takes a long swig and says, "Wow, that's marvelous!"

Then she starts undoing the long zipper that runs down the front of her wetsuit and says, "And how long has it been since you've had some REAL fun?"

"My God!" exclaims the physician, "Don't tell me that you've got golf clubs in there too?"

How many doctors does it take to change a light bulb?
— Only one, but he has to have the nurse tell him which end to screw in.

Why do doctors dress so poorly?
— Drug reps don't give away clothing.

~ DRINKING ~

(See Alcohol)

~ DRUG ABUSE ~

I'm middle aged now. I don't need to do drugs anymore. I can get the same effect just by standing up really fast.
— *Jonathan Katz* [232]

Drugs have taught an entire generation of kids the metric system.
— *P. J. O'Rourke* [235]

~ Drug Representatives ~

I have an idea to help drug companies make money. What if they showed us the same charts and statistics all the time and only changed the names of the drugs as an economy move? *— Homer B. Martin, MD* [199]

On presentations by drug representatives:
Though drug reps are boring,
And their data are crude,
You know you'll keep listening
As long as there's food. *— Michael Hirsch, MD* [167]

Why do doctors dress so poorly?
— Drug reps don't give away clothing.

How many drug reps does it take to change a light bulb?
— Just one, but he has to stand around for an hour until a doctor signs for the bulb.

~ Drugs ~

A drug is a substance that when given to a patient produces the side effect you forgot to mention. *— Howard Bennett, MD* [40]

The desire to take medicine is perhaps the greatest feature that distinguishes man from animals. *— William Osler, MD* [27]

Nowadays there's a pill for everything—to keep your nose from running, to keep your heart beating, to increase your body tone and vigor. Thanks to medical science, people are dying everyday who never looked better.
— Anonymous [234]

Where there's a pill, there's a way. *— Howard Bennett, MD* [36]

Eli Lilly, the pharmaceutical giant, has announced plans to merge with Toys-R-Us. According to a company spokesman, the new company will be called Drugs-R-Us.   — *Larry Bauer, MD* [246]

If you don't know what drug to order, always order the drug on your pen.
— *Rip Pfeiffer, MD* [323]

No doctor's child ever had a disease that could not be adequately treated with whatever was in the drug sample room.   — *David Guttman, MD* [151]

QID is a Latin term. It means, "There's no way I'm taking this pill four times a day."   — *Ryan James, MD* [246]

Balluff's Constant of Memory:
• The number of medications a patient takes are inversely proportional to the patient's ability to remember what those medications are.
• Corollary No. 1: The patient will always describe the medication he cannot remember as "a little white pill."
• Corollary No. 2: If a patient says, "My wife knows what medicines I take," the wife won't have a clue. [101]

A miracle drug is any drug that will do what the label says it will do.
— *Eric Hodgins* [103]

If the whole materia medica, *as now used*, could be sunk to the bottom of the sea, it would be all the better for mankind—and all the worse for the fishes.
— *Oliver Wendell Holmes, MD* [159]

Drug Definitions:
• Elixir: What a dog does to his owner when she gives him a bone.
• Emetic: Someone who drives an ambulance.
• Ester: A girl's name.
• Ether: One or the other.
• Ethyl: Another girl's name.
• Miscible: Not easy to hit.
• Vitamin: What you do when friends stop by for a visit.

A pharmacist handed a medication to an elderly customer and said, "Take one of these every 4 hours, or as often as you can get the cap off."

(See also Antibiotics, Aspirin, Cephalosporins, Compliance, Pharmacists, Placebos)

~ Drug Stores~

Mr. Grubb puffed heavily on his cigar while loitering in a shopping mall drugstore.
The pharmacist said to him, "Please, sir, there's no smoking in the store."
   "But I just bought the cigar here," the man said.
   "Look," the pharmacist said, "we sell laxatives here too, but you can't enjoy them on the premises."

$\mathcal{E}$

~ EAR, NOSE & THROAT ~

A doctor is a person who still has his adenoids, tonsils, and appendix.

— *Laurence J. Peter* [247]

Ear, Nose & Throat Definitions:
• Adenoid: Bothered by drug reps.
• Buccal: Something that holds up your pants.
• Cauterize: What the intern did before he winked at his date.
• Curette: A partial recovery.
• Gland: Chinese for "wonderful."
• Node: Was aware of.
• Orifice: A place of business.
• Serous: Not funny.
• Vertigo: How foreigners ask for directions.

Bloopers & Malapropisms:
• A mother brought her 6-year-old to the office for a throat *sculpture*. (culture)
• Dr. Weissman felt that it was a lymph node and we should sit on it.
• The patient has chronic dizziness due to *blatant* syphilis. (latent)

How many ENTs does it take to change a light bulb?
— None. You don't need it out today, but if it continues to give you trouble in the future you should consider having it removed.

(See also Snoring, Strep Throat)

~ EDUCATION ~

Never try to teach a pig to sing—it wastes your time and it annoys the pig.

— *Paul Dickson* [96]

Doctors and lawyers must go to school for years and years, often with little sleep and with great sacrifice to their first wives. — *Roy Blount, Jr.* [29]

In teaching medical students, the primary requisite is to keep them awake.
— *Chevalier Jackson, MD* [103]

Remember, half the doctors in the country graduated in the bottom half of their class. — *Al McGuire* [135]

Some teachers are born great, some achieve greatness, and some just grate upon you. — *Anonymous* [135]

I have never let my schooling interfere with my education. — *Mark Twain* [19]

Half of what you're taught in medical school will be proven wrong in ten years. The problem is, no one knows which half. — *Anonymous* [103]

As a member of the American Board of Internal Medicine, I tried for six years, unsuccessfully, to get a clinical practice question into the exam to which the correct answer was "nothing." — *Alvan Feinstein, MD* [126]

Comment to William Welch about the entrance standards set for Johns Hopkins Medical School: Welch, it's lucky we got in as professors; we could never get in as students. — *William Osler, MD* [313]

A maiden at college named Breeze
Weighed down by B.A.s and M.D.s
    Collapsed from the strain,
    Said her doctor, "It's plain,
You are killing yourself by degrees!" — *Anonymous* [135]

A professor is one who talks in someone else's sleep. — *W. H. Auden* [298]

(See also Academia, Diploma, Lectures)

~ EKG ~

What do you call two orthopedists reading an EKG?
— A double blind study.

(See also Cardiology, Heart)

~ EMERGENCIES ~

If you can keep your head when all about you are losing theirs, it's possible you haven't grasped the situation. — *Jean Kerr* [172]

Confidence is the feeling you have before you understand the situation. — *Anonymous* [203]

(See also Accidents, Heimlich Maneuver)

~ EMERGENCY MEDICINE ~

If you arrive in the ER and don't know what to do, start putting in tubes until somebody arrives who does. — *Rip Pfeiffer, MD* [248]

ER Slogan: Treat 'em and Street 'em. — *Anonymous* [94]

ER is a great TV show isn't it? After watching a few episodes, you get the feeling that everyone in the country is either bleeding to death or about to. — *Rick Stevens, MD* [246]

Ever go to an emergency room in the South? They're in no hurry down there. I saw a plaque over the door that read, "Time heals all wounds."

— *Judy Gold* [135]

Bloopers & Malapropisms:
• Discharge status: Alive but without permission.
• A 68-year-old asthmatic presented to the emergency room with wheezing and acute shortness of *breast*. (breath)
• The patient's scalp looks pretty bad. The rest of her looks great, however.
• The patient was treated in the emergency room, *X-rated*, and released. (x-rayed)
• He passed a cup of bright red blood per rectum, which brought him to the emergency room.

A 16-year-old went to the emergency room because of a penile discharge and painful urination. He filled out the requisite forms listing his age and address, etc. Under the space that said, "Responsible Party," he wrote, "My girlfriend."

How many ER docs does it take to change a light bulb?
— Just one, but he tries to defibrillate it first.

(See also Cardiac Arrest, First Aid, Heimlich Maneuver, Procedures)

~ ENDOCRINOLOGY ~

A man is as old as his enzymes.

— *James O. Nall, MD* [227]

Being overweight is less often caused by an underactive metabolism than an overactive fork.

— *John G. Hipps, MD* [158]

The human body is a beautiful thing, man, but beauty's only skin deep. Beneath the surface lurks a disgusting and frightening world of guts, gore, and glandular disorders.

— *Bart Simpson* [149]

Bloopers & Malapropisms:
- The patient has an inborn *era* of metabolism. (error)
- This 9-year-old girl was recently diagnosed with a *gross* hormone deficiency. (growth)
- "My doctor diagnosed me with *hashy motor* thyroiditis." (Hashimoto)
- The patient is 68-year-old diabetic who presented with a two week history of *flea-bitus*. (phlebitis)

A doctor looked at the test results for one of his middle-aged patients and was greatly disturbed by what he saw. The man's cholesterol was off the chart, his blood pressure was close to stroke level, and his diabetes was raging out of control. He picked up the phone and called the patient's wife. "I just got your husband's tests back, but I need to speak with you before I give him the results. Your husband is a very sick man and unless you do exactly what I advise, he'll be dead in six months."

"What can I do, doctor?" the woman asked.

"You must remove all sources of stress from his life," the doctor said. "You have to keep the house spotlessly clean, you've got to cook him a nutritious meal three times a day, and you need to have sex with him whenever he asks."

The woman hung up the phone and turned to her husband. "That was Dr. Cama with your lab results," she said.

"What did he say?"

"He says you're gonna die."

How many endocrinologists does it take to change a light bulb?
— Two. One to mix the drinks and the other to call the fellow.

What's the definition of tolerance?
— It's what you get if you give growth hormone to a colony of ants.

(See also Krebs Cycle)

~ ENDOSCOPY ~

Surgeons believe that anything with fiber optics on one end should have a surgeon on the other.   — *Edward Thompson, MD* [305]

Never scope tomorrow what you can scope today.   — *Anonymous* [135]

Endoscopic procedures are invalid unless the patient is naked and hungry.

— John B. Mills, PhD [222]

A new study shows that you can scope all of the people some of the time or some of the people all of the time, but you can't scope all of the people all of the time.

— Howard Bennett, MD [48]

Gastroenterologist to a colleague:
We scoped the patient just in time. In a couple more days he would have gotten better without us.

— Anonymous [137]

(See also Colonoscopy, Gastrointestinal Tract, Procedures, Proctology)

~ EPIDEMIOLOGY ~

An epidemiologist's definition of death:
The ultimate state of the final common pathway that emerges subsequent to a terminal morbid event culminating in the eventual biocessation of animate bio-processes.

— Thomas B. Newman, MD & Warren S. Browner, MD [231]

How many epidemiologists does it take to change a light bulb?
—Six. Three to study the problem of filamentous decay in a population of in-candescent bulbs. Two to write up the report and get it published. And one to call a primary care doc to screw in the new bulb.

~ EPITAPHS ~

(See Last Words)

~ ETHICS ~

An unethical researcher is anyone who gets more grants than you do.

— Howard Bennett, MD [40]

Recognizing the importance of ethical issues in medicine, Dr. Marcus always insisted on the presence of a third party whenever he examined a female patient.

Near the end of a busy afternoon, the doctor wearily motioned a couple into the examination room. The woman complained of pains in her lower abdomen and submitted to a pelvic exam reluctantly. The man looked on with interest.

When he finished, the doctor prescribed some medication and the woman jumped up from the table, dressed hurriedly, and ran from the room.

"Your wife certainly is edgy," the doctor said. "She'll be all right in a few days."

"My wife?" said the man. "I've never seen her before, doc. I was wondering why you called me in here."

A lawyer decided it was time to give his daughter, a recent law school graduate, a lecture on ethics. "In law, ethics are very important," he began. "Suppose, for instance, that a client comes in and settles his $1000 account in cash. After he leaves, you notice an extra $100 stuck to the last bill. Immediately you are presented with an ethical dilemma..." The lawyer paused for dramatic effect, "Should you tell your partner?"

How many ethicists does it take to change a light bulb?
—What makes you think the old bulb wants to be changed?

What's a lawyer's definition of ethics?
— Anything you can get away with.

(See also Doctor-Patient Communication)

~ EXERCISE ~

If God had intended man to engage in strenuous sports, He would have given us better knees.
— *Robert Ray* [62]

My grandmother started walking five miles a day when she was sixty. She's ninety-seven today, and we don't know where the hell she is.
— *Ellen DeGeneris* [96]

If it weren't for the fact that the TV set and the refrigerator are so far apart, some of us wouldn't get any exercise at all. — *Joey Adams* (105)

I believe every human has a finite number of heartbeats. I don't intend to waste any of mine running around doing exercises. — *Neil Armstrong* (15)

I'm pushing 60—that's enough exercise for me. — *Mark Twain* (243)

All that running and exercise can do for you is make you healthy. — *Denny McLain* (62)

Married people don't have to exercise because our attitude is, "They've seen us naked already—and they like it." — *Carol Montgomery* (67)

Have you ever noticed at health clubs that people are always fighting for the closest parking space? — *Anonymous* (135)

Mr. Universe: Don't forget, Mr. Carson, your body is the only home you'll ever have.
Johnny Carson: Yes, my home is pretty messy. But I have a woman who comes in once a week. — *"The Tonight Show"* (217)

I joined a health club last year—spent 400 bucks. Haven't lost a pound. Apparently you have to show up. — *Rich Ceisler* (163)

I'm not into working out. My philosophy—No pain, no pain. — *Carol Leifer* (96)

Whenever I feel like exercise, I lie down until the feeling passes. — *Robert Maynard Hutchens* (191)

(See also Jogging)

~ EXPERIENCE ~

Experience teaches you to recognize a mistake when you've made it again.

— *Anonymous* [135]

Some doctors make the same mistake for twenty years and call it experience.

— *Noah Fabricant, MD* [125]

Experience is what you rely on when you haven't read anything for a while.

— *Howard Bennett, MD* [40]

Napoleon's mules saw a thousand battles, but they were still mules.

— *Anonymous* [191]

Definitions of Clinical Experience:
• "In my experience." *(I have seen one such patient.)*
• "In my series." *(I have seen two such patients.)*
• "In case, after Case, after CASE." *(I have seen three such patients.)*

— *James Dolezal, MD & James Plamadon, MD* [114]

~ EYES ~

(See Ophthalmology)

~ FACE LIFTS ~

A 45-year-old woman who's had a face lift doesn't look twenty-five. If it works, she looks like a well-rested 43-year-old. If it doesn't work, she looks like a Halloween costume.

— Fran Lebowitz [310]

I don't plan to grow old gracefully. I plan to have face-lifts until my ears meet.

— Rita Rudner [245]

~ FAMILY ~

Happiness is having a large, loving, caring, close-knit family—in another city.

— George Burns [88]

A family is a unit composed not only of children, but of men, women, an occasional animal, and the common cold.

— Ogden Nash [249]

Pets are the glue that hold dysfunctional families together.

— Edward Thompson, MD [305]

I love my family, but I hate family reunions. Family reunions are that time when you come face to face with your family tree and realize that some branches need to be cut.

— Rene Hicks [67]

I've been talking about my family with my therapist for so long that by now she has her own problems with these people. Last week, when I was talking about my mother, she said, "Look, I don't want to hear a thing that woman has to say!"

— Sara Cytron [311]

After a good dinner, one can forgive anybody, even one's own relations.

— Oscar Wilde [317]

I take a cold shower every morning—after the rest of my family has taken hot ones.

— Anonymous [218]

~ FAMILY PRACTICE ~

I go to a family physician. He treats my family, and I support his.

— Phyllis Diller [316]

A newspaper ad for a family practice:
Solo practice located in remote wilderness setting. Rugged townsfolk rarely get sick, though you will need to attend to livestock on occasion. Only 1200 miles from a major city and no lawyers in the area.

A surgeon, an internist, and a family practitioner go duck hunting.
    The surgeon sees a duck, shouts, "Duck!" and shoots it down.
    The internist sees a duck, shouts, "Duck! Rule out quail! Rule out pheasant!" and shoots it down.
    The family practitioner sees a duck and blasts it out of the sky with a burst of machine-gun fire. As the tattered carcass falls to the ground, he remarks, "I don't know what the hell it was, but I sure got it."

(For a variation on this joke, see page 197.)

How many family practitioners does it take to change a light bulb?
— Just one, but the bulb will have to spend two hours in the waiting room.

(See also Generalist, Medical Practice, PMDs, Primary Care)

~ FAT ~

(See Cholesterol)

~ Fatherhood ~

My daughter has me totally wrapped around her little finger. I don't even try to win anymore. I just try to save face. I say things like, "Go to your room at your earliest convenience, okay? Daddy's going to count to fifteen hundred."

— Jonathan Katz [(232)]

Fathers should neither be seen nor heard. That is the only proper basis for family life.

— Oscar Wilde [(318)]

On baby intercoms:
She's in the crib with one part of the intercom and I'm in the other room. "Breaker one-nine. Daddy, I got spitup on my shirt and I'm packing a load. Please come in and help me."

— Bob Saget [(135)]

(See also Babies, Children, Motherhood, Parenting)

~ Fatigue ~

A woman goes to her doctor complaining that she is tired all of the time. After the diagnostic tests show nothing, the doctor asks her how often she has intercourse.

"Every Monday, Wednesday, and Saturday," she says.

The doctor advises her to cut out Wednesdays.

"I can't," the woman says. "That's the only night I'm home with my husband."

~ Fees ~

(See Bills)

~ Fever ~

If you don't take a temperature, you won't find a fever.

— Anonymous [(94)]

A fever is a change in body temperature that decreases a doctor's sleep, but increases his income.
— *Howard Bennett, MD* [46]

Fever spike: Something that happens the night before a patient is scheduled for nursing home placement.
— *Rip Pfeiffer, MD* [248]

Small fevers gratefully accepted.
— *Oliver Wendell Holmes, Sr., MD (attrib.)* [135]

(See also Infectious Disease)

~ FIRST AID ~

I've already had medical attention—a dog licked me when I was on the ground.
— *Neil Simon* [288]

One hot summer afternoon, a man fainted in the middle of a busy intersection. As traffic began to back up, a woman rushed to help him. As she knelt down to loosen his collar, a man emerged from the crowd, pushed her aside, and said, "It's all right, honey, I've taken a course in first aid."

The woman stood up and watched as the man took the victim's pulse and prepared to administer rescue breathing. Then she tapped him on the shoulder.

"When you get to the part about calling a doctor," she said, "I'm already here."

Jody was telling her friends how the first aid course she took had prepared her for an emergency earlier in the day.

"I saw this accident where a pedestrian was hit by a car. His arm was broken, and his face was covered with blood."

"So what did you do?" her friends asked.

"Thanks to the first aid course, I knew exactly what to do—I sat down on the curb and put my head between my knees to keep from fainting."

(See also Accidents, Emergencies, Heimlich Maneuver)

~ FLATUS ~

My sister-in-law had a lot of gas when she was pregnant with her first child. One night was particularly eventful so I said, "Laura, would you mind going into another room until you're done?" She said, "If I left the room every time I had to pass gas, I'd never be here."

— *Howard Bennett, MD* [48]

When I sat by the duchess at tea,
It was just as I knew it would be,
   Her rumblings abdominal
   Were really phenomenal;
And everyone thought it was me.

— *William Bennett Bean, MD* [28]

Dr. Johnson, when sober or pissed,
Could be frequently heard to insist
   Letting out a great fart:
   "Yes, I follow Descartes—
I stink, and I therefore exist."

— *Anonymous* [241]

There once was a patient named White
Who always called doctors at night.
   His problem was flatus,
   His family said, "Save us!"
But no one could undo his plight.

— *Larry Bauer, MD* [246]

~ FOOD ~

Part of the secret of success in life is to eat what you like and let the food fight it out inside.

— *Mark Twain* [191]

My kids will only eat three foods and two of them are macaroni and cheese.

— *Rachel Ruina* [246]

To eat is human. To digest, divine.

— *Charles T. Copeland* [298]

Food is an important part of a balanced diet.

— *Fran Lebowitz* [103]

Red meat is not bad for you. Now blue-green meat, *that's* bad for you.
— *Tommy Smothers* [135]

Vegetables are substances used by children to balance their plate while carrying it to and from the dining table. — *Anonymous* [134]

An old maxim is, "If you eat slowly, you will eat less." This is particularly true if you're a member of a large family. — *Anonymous* [135]

You do live longer with bran, but you spend the last fifteen years in the bathroom. — *Alan King* [322]

(See also Dieting, Health Food, Obesity, Vegetarians)

~ FOREIGN BODY ~

A foreign body is any object smaller than a toaster that is left in the vicinity of a young child for less than two minutes. — *Howard Bennett, MD* [46]

A frantic father called his pediatrician late one night. "Please hurry," he said, "my 4-year-old just swallowed a ballpoint pen."
    "I'll be there in 20 minutes," said the doctor.
    "What should I do until you get here?" the father wanted to know.
    "Use a pencil."

A nurse called a resident at 3 AM. "Come quick," she said. "Your patient, Mrs. Parks, just swallowed a thermometer."
    The resident hung up the phone and put on his jacket, but before he could get out the door the nurse called back.
    "Never mind," she said. "I found another one."

~ FRACTURES ~

A child's fracture will heal if both ends of the bone are in the same room.
— *Anonymous* [248]

When I was younger, if any of us kids got sick, my mother would bring out the chicken soup. Of course, that didn't work for broken bones. For broken bones, she gave us boiled beef.

— George Burns [242]

~ FREUD ~

A Freudian slip is when you say one thing but mean your mother.

— Anonymous [135]

Sometimes a cigar is just a cigar.

— Sigmund Freud [94]

An early psychiatrist, Freud,
Had the *bluenoses* very annoyed,
   Saying, "You cannot be rid
   Of the troublesome Id,
So it might just as well be enjoyed."

— Anonymous [85]

According to old Sigmund Freud,
Life is seldom so well enjoyed
   As in human coition
   (In any position)
With the usual organs employed.

— Anonymous [241]

After three years in analysis, a patient had her last therapy session with Sigmund Freud. On leaving the office, the patient turned to the celebrated doctor with a puzzled look on her face. Noting her expression, Freud said, "Do you have a question my dear?"

"Why yes, Herr Freud, I do. After all these years in therapy, I'm still not sure what a phallus is."

At this point, Freud escorted the woman back into his office, pulled down his trousers and pointed between his legs. "This, my dear, is a phallus."

"Oh, I see," said the patient. "It's like a penis . . . only smaller."

How many Freudians does it take to change a light bulb?
— Two. One to hold the ladder and the other to change the penis. Oops! I mean, bulb.

"Is it true that Natalie's son is seeing a psychiatrist?" a woman asked her friend.

"That's what I heard," she answered.

"So what's his problem?"

"The doctor says that he has a severe Oedipus complex."

"Oedipus-schmedipus—as long as he loves his mother."

(See also Psychiatry, Psychoanalysis)

G

~ GALLBLADDER ~

One of the most difficult things to contend with in a hospital is the assumption on the part of the staff that because you have lost your gallbladder you have also lost your mind. — *Jean Kerr* [172]

A gallbladder is what you have taken out before the doctor decides it's an ulcer. — *Anonymous* [124]

A woman with abdominal pain goes to see the doctor. After a brief examination, the doctor tells her she has inflamed gallstones and needs an operation right away. The woman decides to get another opinion. The second doctor tells her she has indigestion and heart trouble. "I'm going back to the first doctor," the woman says. "I'd rather have gallstones."

~ GAS ~

(See Flatus)

~ GASTROINTESTINAL TRACT ~

I have finally come to the conclusion that a good, reliable set of bowels is worth more to a man than any quantity of brains. — *Josh Billings* [125]

Comment about a patient with years of imaginary bowel complaints:
When I die, it will not be my life which flashes before my eyes, but Mrs. P's bowel—all twenty feet of it. And it will not flash, but glide by majestically, enabling me to examine it all in painful detail. And it will look entirely normal. — *Keith Hopcraft, MD* [162]

Diaphragm, n. A muscular partition separating disorders of the chest from disorders of the bowels.

— *Ambrose Bierce* [51]

The general practitioner's association with the bowels begins with the digestion of large amounts of information in medical school. Quite often this intellectual nutrition is in a high fiber form; much of it is unabsorbed and goes straight through.

— *J. Dowden, MD* [115]

Gastrointestinal Definitions:
• Alimentary: What Sherlock Holmes said to Dr. Watson.
• Bowel: A letter like a-e-i-o-u.
• Innuendo: Where an Italian gastroenterologist puts his proctoscope.
• Orifice: A place of business.
• Rectum: What being up all night did to the intern.

Bloopers & Malapropisms:
• Both the patient and the nurse herself reported passing flatus.
• The patient presents with a history of intermittent *tardy* stools. (tarry)
• The patient was examined with a *well-challenged* sigmoidoscope. (Welch-Allyn)
• The patient was diagnosed in 1994 with *all-sorts-of-colitis*. (ulcerative colitis)
• He has a long history of *portable* hypertension. (portal)
• The patient's bleeding started in the rectal area and continued all the way to Los Angeles.
• Drinking is a major cause of *psoriasis* of the liver. (cirrhosis)
• Ever since Mrs. Wilson had her gallbladder removed, she can't tolerate greasy *males*. (meals)
• The patient stated that she was constipated for most of her life until 1998 when she got divorced.

(See also Colon, Colonoscopy, Constipation, Diarrhea, Endoscopy, Flatus, Hepatitis, Hiccups, Indigestion, Pancreas, Ulcers, Vomiting)

~ GENERALIST ~

A generalist is someone who learns less and less about more and more until he knows nothing about everything. A specialist is someone who learns more and more about less and less until he knows everything about nothing.

— *Anonymous* [94]

The primary goal of all generalists is to save patients from specialists.

— Anonymous [94]

(See also Family Practice, PMDs, Specialists)

~ GENETICS ~

Scientists have found the gene for shyness. They would have found it years ago, but it was hiding behind a couple of other genes. *— Jonathan Katz* [232]

A wife complains to her husband about his irresponsible brother:
Barbara: I can't believe you two are from the same gene pool.
Mitch: He's from the shallow end. *— "City Slickers II"* [91]

On the long time it takes for genetics to affect a population:
Anything even remotely connected with genetics takes forever. Even a single medical school lecture on genetics takes years to end. *— Mark DePaolis, MD* [109]

All modern men are descended from worm-like creatures, but it shows more on some people. *— Will Cuppy* [194]

Genetic Definitions:
• Genotype: The type of girl Gino likes.
• Inbred: The best way to eat bologna.

(See also Cloning, Heredity)

~ GERIATRICS ~

My research friends tell me that they have difficulty evaluating the quality of life in the elderly. There are three features one has to deal with—one is work, another is play, and the third is sex. The problem with the elderly is they don't know whether to classify sex as work or play. *— William Kannel, MD* [171]

(See also Nursing Homes, Old Age, VA Hospitals)

~ GLASSES ~

Now that I'm over fifty, I have to hold the newspaper a little farther from my face every year. It's not that my eyes aren't strong enough. It's just that my arms aren't long enough.

— *Anonymous* [135]

Men seldom make passes
At girls who wear glasses.

— *Dorothy Parker* [298]

Yesterday I was walking down the street wearing my glasses when all of a sudden my prescription ran out.

— *Steven Wright* [139]

(See also Ophthalmology)

~ GOUT ~

If you drink wine you will have the gout, and if you do not drink wine the gout will have you.

— *Thomas Sydenham* [298]

I have gout, asthma, and seven other maladies, but am otherwise very well.

— *Sydney Smith* [298]

On patients with gout:
Those who suffer so afflicted
Colchicined and Benemided,
Have my heartfelt sympathy;
Thanks to God it's them not me.

— *A. Nathan Caplan, MD* [81]

A patient wasn't sure whether he had rheumatism or gout. He asked his doctor what the difference was.

The doctor answered, "Suppose you put your thumb in a vise and screw it so tight that you can not longer endure the pain. That's rheumatism. Now, give the vise one more turn. That's gout."

(See also Arthritis)

~ GRAND ROUNDS ~

Sitting through Grand Rounds is like eating a plate of vegetables—you know it's good for you, but you'd rather have fries.   — *Howard Bennett, MD* [40]

There's nothing wrong with Grand Rounds that a little Valium won't fix.
— *Anonymous* [135]

By a speaker at Grand Rounds:
I don't mind if you look at your watches, but when you hold them up to your ears, that hurts my feelings.   — *Anonymous* [203]

A well-known allergist was scheduled to give Grand Rounds at a local hospital. As he was about to leave his secretary said, "Dr. Keating, I've heard this lecture so many times, I bet I could do it myself. Why don't you rest at the back of the auditorium while I give the talk?"

Since the doctor had been up all night with a sick patient, he agreed.

At the hospital, the allergist settled into the back row for a rest while his secretary gave the lecture. At the end of the talk, the secretary asked if there were any questions.

"Yes," said one doctor, who proceeded to ask a rather difficult question.

The secretary got nervous, but recovered quickly and said, "That's such an easy question, I'm going to let my secretary answer it."

~ GRANTS ~

An unethical researcher is anyone who gets more grants than you do.
— *Howard Bennett, MD* [48]

(See also Research)

~ GYNECOLOGY ~

Going to a male gynecologist is like going to an auto mechanic who never owned a car.   — *Carrie Snow* [168]

I'm not much of a Southern belle. Southern women tend to be real demure. They don't like to talk about anything graphic. I had a girlfriend who told me she was in the hospital for female problems. I said, "What does that mean?" She says, "You know, female problems." I said, "What? You can't parallel park? You can't get credit?"

— *Pam Stone* [23]

On asking kids what their dads do for a living:
My dad is a gynecologist. He looks at vaginas all day long.

— *"Kindergarten Cop"* [177]

I got a postcard from my gynecologist. It said, "Did you know it's time for you annual check-up?" No, but now my mailman does. — *Cathy Ladman* [310]

On going out with gynecologists:
Never date a man who knows more about your vagina than you do.

— *Dana Stevens* [135]

Bloopers & Malapropisms:
• The pelvic exam will be done later on the floor.
• The speculum was inserted between the *eyes.* (os)
• Past medical history reveals that the patient was admitted two years ago with a *Bavarian* cyst. (ovarian)
• She was treated with Mycostatin oral *suppositories.* (suspension)
• The patient is a 48-year-old woman who was seen for a *screaming* mammogram. (screening)
• Dr. Robinson has been following the patient's breast for six months.
• "I need to make an appointment for my annual *Pabst* smear." (pap)
• After suffering from heavy menstrual periods, the 54-year-old patient asked if she would need a *resurrectomy.* (hysterectomy)
• The patient had a pelvic ultrasound to rule out an *overbearing* cyst. (ovarian)

What are the four most common OB/GYN procedures?
• Removing female organs.
• Repairing female organs.
• Cutting the left ureter (oops).
• Cutting the right ureter (oops, again).

What did the gynecologist say to his patient?
— I'm at your cervix.

Mary O'Toole lived in a small town her whole life and had always been as healthy as a horse. Unfortunately, as middle age approached, she found herself suffering from some "female" trouble. She told her daughter-in-law about the problem, who called a gynecologist and drove her to the appointment.

A wide-eyed Mrs. O'Toole lay still as a stone as the doctor examined her. When it was over, she looked up and said, "You seem like such a nice young man. But tell me, does your mother know what you do for a living?"

After 15 years as an OB/GYN, a doctor decided it was time to change careers. He pondered his options for a few weeks until he remembered how much he enjoyed automotive class in high school. So the doctor enrolled at a local automotive school. Upon completion of the course, his final exam consisted of taking a car engine apart and putting it back together. The doctor took the exam and, to his astonishment, received a grade of 150%. After class, he said to his instructor, "You know, I've turned in plenty of perfect papers in my life, but how does one get a score of 150%?"

"Well," the instructor replied. "I gave you 50% for taking the engine apart and 50% for putting it back together. The other 50% was because you did it all through the tailpipe."

How many gynecologists does it take to change a light bulb?
— None. They'd say, "Why not take out the whole socket? You're not using it, and it will only cause you trouble in the future."

(See also Mammograms, Menopause, Menstruation, Obstetrics, Pelvic Exam, PMS, Uterus, Vagina)

ℋ

~ HABITS ~

Nothing so needs reforming as other people's habits. — *Mark Twain* [19]

A behavioral psychologist is someone who pulls habits out of rats.
— *Douglas Busch, PhD* [247]

~ HANDICAPS ~

I'm proud to be handicapped. If it weren't for me you'd be spending all day looking for a place to park. — *Gene Mitchner* [84]

Recently, in a public bathroom, I used the handicapped stall. As I emerged, a man in a wheelchair asked me indignantly, "Are you handicapped?" Gathering all my aplomb, I looked him in the eye and said, "Not now, but I was before I went in there." — *George Carlin* [67]

~ HEADACHES ~

When I get headaches, I do what it says on the aspirin bottle—Take two, and keep away from children. — *Roseanne Barr* [135]

Never have a headache on the same day as your husband; but if you do, be sure to mention it first. — *E. V. Lucas* [124]

Mr. Chase was having terrible headaches, so he called his doctor for an appointment.
    "I can squeeze you in next week," the receptionist said.
    "Next week? Lady, I could be dead by then."
    "In that case," she said, "please have someone call and cancel the appointment."

A man with a long history of migraines goes to see a neurologist. During the history and physical examination, the doctor discovers that the patient hasn't responded to any of the standard treatments for his condition.

"Listen," the doc says, "I have migraines too and the advice I'm going to give you can't be found in any medical book, but it has served me well over the years. When I get a migraine I go home, take a hot bath, and put a cold washcloth on my forehead. Then I get out of the tub, go to the bedroom, and make passionate love to my wife. Almost always, the headache is gone immediately. Now, give it a try and see me in a month or so."

Six weeks later, the patient returns for a follow-up visit. "Doc, I took your advice and it works. It really works! This is the first time in seventeen years that anything has helped my headaches."

"Well," the neurologist says, "I'm glad I could help."

"By the way, Doc," the patient adds. "You have a really nice house."

(See also Aspirin, Neurology)

~ Health ~

The only way to keep your health is to eat what you don't want, drink what you don't like, and do things you'd rather not. — *Mark Twain* [298]

If you've got your health, you've got everything. And if you don't have your health, sooner or later your doctor has everything. — *Gene Perret* [243]

Telling someone he looks healthy isn't a compliment—it's a second opinion. — *Fran Lebowitz* [135]

It's no longer a question of staying healthy. It's a question of finding a sickness you like. — *Jackie Mason* [135]

When it comes to my health, I think of my body as a temple . . . or at least a moderately well-run Presbyterian Youth Center. — *Emo Philips* [163]

Health—what my friends are always drinking to before they fall down. — *Phyllis Diller* [310]

Since I came to the White House, I got two hearing aids, a colon operation, skin cancer, a prostate operation, and I was shot. The damn thing is, I've never felt better in my life.   — *Ronald Reagan* [323]

Quit worrying about your health. It'll go away.   — *Robert Orben* [186]

(See also Exercise, Wellness)

~ HEALTH CARE BOOKS ~

Be careful about reading health books. You may die of a misprint.
                                                                  — *Mark Twain* [19]

Calories do count,
Dear Dr. Taller;
I followed your book
And I'm not any smaller.   — *Marian Bigwood* [52]

On birth control:
Sister Susie built her hopes
On the books of Mary Stopes.
But I fear from her condition,
She must have read the wrong edition.   — *Madge Kendall* [98]

(See also Self Help)

~ HEALTH CARE COSTS ~

The underlying philosophy of our entire health care system is that the more scary, painful, dangerous, and unnecessary a medical procedure is, the more it should cost.   — *Dave Barry* [26]

Why does the general internist need new specialized technological procedures? He needs to use a colonoscope to be able to extract the $800 bill that's up there.   — *Alvan Feinstein, MD* [126]

My computer caught a health care virus. It goes through your system for hours, finds nothing wrong, and sends you a bill for $2,500.   — *Anonymous* [135]

(See also Bills)

~ HEALTH CARE REFORM ~

Los Angeles can be a strange place to live. My car was recently forced off the road by aliens. I was extricated from the vehicle and led on board the mothership, where I was subjected to an extensive battery of excruciatingly painful anal probes. And as I lay on the workbench and begged for my life, the head alien tried to assuage my fears by reassuring me that most, if not all, of the tests would hopefully be covered under Clinton's comprehensive health care package.
— *Dennis Miller* [139]

Money has become such a big issue at medical centers, that the phrase *primum non nocere* will no longer be taught to medical students. From now on, the first rule of medicine will be *primum no dinero*.   — *Howard Bennett, MD* [39]

A new movie just opened called *The Fugitive*. It's about a doctor who is on the run. Guess he must have gotten a look at Clinton's health plan.   — *Jay Leno* [135]

If health care becomes nationalized, we'll get a system with the compassion of the Internal Revenue Service and the efficiency of the Post Office.
— *Louis Sullivan, MD* [299]

It's impossible to go anywhere these days without getting into a discussion about health care reform. It happens at conferences. It happens at PTA meetings. It even happens when you're standing in line at the men's room. Not that health care reform isn't an important issue. It's just that sometimes the burning desire to cure the nation's ills takes a back seat to the burning desire to empty one's bladder.   — *Howard Bennett, MD* [39]

~ HEALTH FOOD ~

Health food makes me sick.   — *Calvin Trillin* [249]

Personally, I stay away from health foods. At my age, I need all the preservatives I can get. *— George Burns* [243]

Have you ever seen the customers in health-food stores? They are pale, skinny people who look half dead. In a steak house, you see robust, ruddy people. They're dying, of course, but they look terrific. *— Bill Cosby* [135]

Health food nuts are going to feel stupid someday, lying in hospitals dying of nothing. *— Red Foxx* [134]

Scientists don't know what's in tofu because even they're afraid to touch it. *— Paula Poundstone* [135]

I have a friend who's a macrobiotic. She doesn't eat meat, chicken, fish, white flour, sugar, or preservatives. She's pale, sickly, and exhausted just from looking for something to eat. *— Paula Poundstone* [135]

(See also Food, Vegetarians)

~ HEALTH INSURANCE ~

I recently became a Christian Scientist. It was the only health plan I could afford. *— Betsy Salkind* [186]

On limiting days in the hospital after having a baby:
Naturally, these decisions are all made by men, who have no idea what it feels like to deliver a baby. Women know that any male who passed a seven-pound object through his own reproductive organs would be in intensive care for months, besides receiving years of therapy afterward. *— Mark DePaolis, MD* [109]

Have you ever noticed that people take poetic license with their use of the title Doctor? Pick up any *Yellow Pages* and you'll find Bike Doctors, Rug Doctors, Lawn Doctors, and even Drain Doctors. I wonder what happens if your rug gets sick in the middle of the night? "Is this the Rug Doctor? Yes, my 4-year-old just spilled some Hawaiian Punch on our $2,000 oriental rug. No, we don't have rug insurance . . . Hello?" *— Howard Bennett, MD* [48]

President Clinton signed a bill that requires insurance companies to let mothers stay a minimum of 48 hours after their baby is born. To qualify, all the mother has to do is sign a form swearing that Bill Clinton isn't the father.

— *Jay Leno* [135]

High insurance rates are what really killed the dinosaurs. — *David Letterman* [135]

Milton Bradley just came out with a new board game. It's called "Health Care Deluxe." Players move around the board getting various diseases, paying insurance premiums, and making appointments to see doctors. The problem is, whenever you pick a Treatment Card, they all say CLAIM DENIED!

— *Rick Stevens, MD* [246]

With health insurance, people who smoke and eat pork rinds pay the same rate as marathon runners. Your only reward for taking care of yourself is that you live longer, which allows you to pay more premiums. — *Mark DePaolis, MD* [108]

A woman calls her insurance company to find out what her benefits are now that she is pregnant. Her agent says, "I'm sorry, Mrs. Wright, but your policy only pays for sickness and accidents."

"This was an accident," she answers.

Did you hear about the terrorist who hijacked a plane full of insurance executives on their way to a convention? He threatened to release one every hour if his demands weren't met.

How many doctors does it take to change a light bulb?
— That depends on what type of health insurance it has.

(See also Managed Care)

~ HEARING LOSS ~

My grandmother's ninety and she's dating again. He's ninety-three. It's going great. They never argue—they can't hear each other. — *Cathy Ladman* [184]

A 92-year-old man went to see his doctor for a physical. A few days later, the doctor saw the man walking down the street with a beautiful young woman on his arm.

The following week, the old man went back to the doctor to get his test results. "You're really doing great aren't you?" the doctor said.

"Just following orders, doc," the old man replied. "Like you said, 'Get a hot mama and be cheerful'."

"I didn't say that," the doctor announced. "I said you had a heart murmur and told you to be careful."

On his 90th birthday, a man gets a surprise party from his friends. Halfway through the party, they wheel in a big birthday cake and out pops a beautiful young woman who says, "Hi, Ben, would you like some super sex?"

The man says, "Well, I guess I'll take the soup."

A man goes to his doctor and complains that his wife can't hear.

"How bad is it?" the doctor asks.

"I have no idea," the husband answers.

"Well," the doctors says, "what you need to do is test her. Say something from far away and then repeat it as you get closer. Once she hears you, we'll have an idea what her range of hearing is."

So the man goes home and finds his wife preparing something in the kitchen. From 20 feet away: "What are we having for dinner?" No answer.

From 10 feet: Same thing.

From 5 feet: Same thing.

Finally, the man stands right behind his wife and says, "So, what's for dinner?"

She turns around, looks him in the face, and says, "For the FOURTH time, we're having BEEF STEW!"

(See also Nursing Homes, Old Age)

~ HEART ~

Except for an occasional heart attack, I feel as young as I ever did.

— *Robert Benchley* [74]

The really bad thing about the heart is the sex thing. See, you gotta be careful about sex now. You get that heart pumping and suddenly, boom! Next thing you know you got a hose coming out of your chest attached to a piece of luggage.

— *Kramer, "Seinfeld"* [276]

Heart, n. (orthopedic definition) A muscular organ whose sole purpose is to pump blood to the bones.
— *Anonymous* [94]

Medical science is making advances every day to control health problems. In fact, it's probably only a matter of time before a heart attack, you know, becomes like a headache. We'll just see people on TV going, "I had a heart attack . . . but I gave myself one of these (puts electrode paddles to chest) . . . Brrhht . . . and it's gone."
— *Jerry Seinfeld* [275]

On the early use of beta-blockers in heart attack patients:
I don't think I would give a beta-blocker to somebody who came in with bronchospasm, a blood pressure of 70, pulmonary edema, and a heart rate of 50. Particularly if his lawyer was with him.
— *Adolph Hutter, MD* [164]

When the nurse came to give Mrs. Johnson her heart medication, the patient looked skeptically at the pills.

"Excuse me," the patient said, "but I was just reading about a woman who checked into a hospital for heart trouble, and she ended up dying because the nurse gave her the wrong medicine."

The nurse smiled. "Rest easy, Mrs. Johnson. When a patient comes in here with heart trouble, she *dies* of heart trouble."

A 70-year-old man married a younger woman. After five years of a very happy marriage, he had a heart attack. The doctor advised him that to prolong his life he needed to cut out the sex.

The man and his wife discussed the problem and decided that he would sleep in the family room downstairs to save them both from temptation.

One night, several weeks later, he decided that life without sex wasn't worth living, so he headed upstairs. He met his wife on the staircase and said, "I was coming up to die."

She laughed and replied, "I was coming down to kill you."

(See also Cardiology, Chest Pain)

~ HEARTBURN ~

(See Indigestion)

~ HEIMLICH MANEUVER ~

I had to do the Heimlich Maneuver in a French restaurant the other night. When it was over, the guy said, "Doc, what can I do to thank you?" I looked over at his table and said, "Stop eating filet mignon with cheap red wine."

— *Larry Bauer, MD* [246]

A man at a restaurant suddenly began choking on a piece of steak. His face grew redder and redder as the other diners watched, not knowing what to do. Finally, someone rushed over and said, "I'm a doctor. Let me help." The doctor did a Heimlich maneuver and the meat shot out of the man's mouth.

The grateful diner turned to the doctor and said, "Thank you for saving my life. Now tell me, how much do I owe you?"

The doctor said, "I'll settle for half of what you would have given me two minutes ago."

(See also Emergencies, First Aid)

~ HEMATOLOGY ~

Bloopers & Malapropisms:
• The patient takes iron for a low *hemogoblin*. (hemoglobin)
• The patient was transfused with two units of blood in order to decrease his symptoms. The SOB was the same on discharge, however.
• Examination of the extremities revealed petechiae and *ickymoses*. (ecchymoses)

(See also Blood & Blood Drawing, Iron Deficiency, Spleen)

~ HEMORRHOIDS ~

On sphincter protecting hemorrhoidectomies:
The sphincter ani is like the goalie in hockey—always alert. It can tell whether its owner is alone or with someone, whether standing up or sitting down, whether its owner has his pants on or off . . . a muscle like that is worth protecting.

— *William Bornemeier, MD* [60]

Hemorrhoid, n. Transportation afforded a third person; as, "He didn't have his car so I offered hemorrhoid."
— *H. S. Grannatt* [144]

Is it really necessary to print "USE ONLY AS DIRECTED" on a tube of hemorrhoid cream?
— *Lewis Grizzard* [148]

Hemorrhoids are the body's revenge for a high fat diet.
— *Anonymous* [135]

If you've seen one hemorrhoid, you've seen them all.
— *Anonymous* [135]

If a guy films his wife giving birth, she ought to be able to film his hemorrhoid surgery later on—"Look girls, Tony is totally dilated. What a trouper he was."
— *Jeff Foxworthy* [135]

From the Hemorrhoid Hotline:
Are you afraid to sit on the john? Are you troubled that your next stool may be your last? Don't suffer alone! Our trained volunteers are standing by 24 hours a day. Call now: 1-800-SCRATCH.

Dr. March was on his way back from a lecture when he stopped at a diner for a late night snack. While studying the menu, he looked up and noticed the waitress was scratching at her rear end. "You got hemorrhoids?" the doctor inquired.
   "Sorry, no special orders," the waitress said. "Just what's on the menu."

~ HEPATITIS ~

It has been estimated that the chance of acquiring hepatitis from oysters is about 1 in 10,000; therefore, no more than 9,999 of these delicacies should be consumed in one sitting.
— *Stanley L Robbins, MD* [260]

(See also Liver)

~ HEREDITY ~

Heredity is what sets the parents of a teenager wondering about each other.
— *Laurence J. Peter* [105]

The law of heredity is that all undesirable traits come from the other parent.
— *Anonymous* [103]

A child's definition of heredity:
If your grandfather didn't have any children, and your father didn't have any children, then the chances are you won't have any either.

(See also Genetics)

~ HERNIAS ~

There was a young man with a hernia
Who said to his doctor, "Gol-dernya!
   When carving my middle
   Be sure you don't fiddle
With matters that do not concernya."
— *Heywood Broun* [116]

I never tell people that I'm a doctor when I make dinner reservations. Sure, I may get a table near the kitchen, but at least I won't get stuck listening to the maitre d' tell me about his upcoming hernia operation.   — *Molly Ryan, MD* [246]

From a medical student's note:
The patient was referred for evaluation of *bilingual* hernias. (inguinal)

A sexy young woman had surgery for an inguinal hernia. After the operation, her surgeon stopped by to see how she was doing. "I'm doing very well, Dr. Hartman, but I was wondering if the scar will show?"
   "My dear," replied the doctor, "that is entirely up to you."

~ Hiccups ~

A man rushed into a drug store and said to the pharmacist, "Do you have anything that will stop hiccups?"

The pharmacist leaned over the counter and slapped the man in the face.

"Why the heck did you do that?" the man said.

"It stopped your hiccups didn't it?"

"I don't have the hiccups, you dumbbell. My wife does, and she's in the car."

~ High Blood Pressure ~

A friend I know could never remember his blood pressure, but said that if his diastolic reading was under his golf score, he was happy.   — *Erma Bombeck* [135]

~ Hippocrates ~

A spoof on his aphorisms:
• Absence of respiration is a bad sign.
• It is unfavorable for the patient to be purple, especially if he is also cold. The physician should not promise a cure in such cases.
• When the spleen is found on the right side, the patient should consider changing physicians.
• The surgeon requires a steady hand and a calm disposition. It is also essential to have a patient.
• In patients who are filled with nothing but crude humors, removal of all the blood relieves the symptoms.
• Where symptoms are protracted it is good (for the physician) if the patient's relatives are few, and best if they be absent altogether.
• The physician should not condemn ancient medicine merely because it was ineffective. The Art is eternal.   — *S. N. Gaño, MD* [136]

Money has become such a big issue at medical centers, that the phrase *primum non nocere* will no longer be taught to medical students. From now on, the first rule of medicine will be *primum no dinero*.   — *Howard Bennett, MD* [39]

~ History & Physical Examination ~

If all else fails, do an H&P.

— *Anonymous* [94]

Deferred, adj. Refers to part of the physical exam that was not done on admission. It's not likely to be done after admission either.

— *Faith T. Fitzgerald, MD* [127]

Oriented X Three: A patient who is less confused than his physician.

— *Anonymous* [94]

The key thing to remember during a history and physical is not to tell the doctor what you think is wrong. Doctors hate this. They went to school for seven or eight years, and they like to put this medical training to use:

Doctor: What's wrong?
Patient: I think I fractured my arm.
Doctor: What makes you think that?
Patient: Well, I have a new elbow where the bowling ball hit it.
Doctor: Now, let's not jump to conclusions. First we'll have to run some tests, maybe a controlled study on the other arm. Nurse, bring me a bowling ball, please.

— *Mark DePaolis, MD* [110]

An intern was taking a history on a new patient in the clinic. "You seem to be in excellent health, Mrs. Malloy. Could you tell me what your parents died of?"

"I can't remember," the patient answered. "But I'm sure it was nothing serious."

Bloopers and Malapropisms:
• The intern's admission note revealed that "the patient was unresponsive in bed."
• The patient has no past history of suicides.
• Coming from Detroit, this man has no children.
• Rectal exam revealed a normal sized thyroid.
• The patient has two teenage children, but no other abnormalities.
• The patient was alert and unresponsive.
• The patient is an 82-year-old widow who no longer lives with her husband.
• The patient had waffles for breakfast and anorexia for lunch.

- When she fainted, her eyes rolled around the room.
- While in the ER, she was examined, *X-rated*, and sent home. (x-rayed)
- "My wife has had stomachaches for the past six months, but I think they're *psychoceramic*. (psychosomatic)

(See also Physical Diagnosis, Symptoms)

~ HMOs ~

(See Managed Care)

~ HOMEOPATHY ~

A homeopathist is someone who has nothing and wants to share it with the world.
— *Anonymous* [135]

How many homeopathists does it take to change a light bulb?
— Just one, but it takes six months to do it.

(See also Acupuncture, Chiropractor)

~ HOSPITAL ADMINISTRATION ~

No one knows what hospital administrators do, but it evidently requires beautiful offices full of Scandinavian teak furniture.
— *Mark DePaolis, MD* [110]

You know you're a physician executive if:
- Your pen is more expensive than your stethoscope.
- Other physicians don't understand your abbreviations.
- The term "managed care" gets you excited.
— *Joshua H. Bennett, MD* [49]

Hospital administrators should be seen and not heard.
— *Anonymous* [135]

Guidelines for Administrators:
• When in charge, ponder.
• When in trouble, delegate.
• When in doubt, mumble.
— *James H. Boren* [322]

Epstein's Law: If you think the problem is bad now, just wait until we've solved it. [135]

~ HOSPITALS ~

One of the most difficult things to contend with in a hospital is the assumption on the part of the staff that because you have lost your gallbladder you have also lost your mind.
— *Jean Kerr* [172]

A hospital bed is a parked taxi with the meter running.
— *Groucho Marx* [29]

Taylor's Law: If they can sign out AMA, they must be alive. [135]

Why is it better to be a doctor than a patient? There's a better chance you'll leave the hospital alive.
— *Anne Eva Ricks, MD* [256]

On problems with getting the right hospital supplies:
When I order rectal thermometers, I get spark plugs. Both useful items, but hardly interchangeable.
— *Colonel Potter, "M*A*S*H"* [200]

There are two types of people who work in hospitals—those who think medical students are a pain in the butt and those who want to date them.
— *Howard Bennett, MD* [48]

An elderly woman went to the hospital to visit a friend. She hadn't been in a hospital for years and felt nervous about all the new technology. A technician followed her onto the elevator wheeling a large machine with lots of tubes and dials.

"Boy, I'd hate to be hooked up to that thing," she said.

"So would I," replied the technician. "It's our new carpet cleaner."

"We need to get this man to the hospital right away," the doctor said to his receptionist.

"What is it?"

"It's a big building with lots of doctors, but that's not important now."

How many hospital employees does it take to change a light bulb?
— Sorry, due to cost containment, that item has been cut from the budget.

(See also Nurses, Patients & Patient Care, VA Hospitals, Ward Clerks)

~ HOUSE CALLS ~

The best way to get a doctor to make a house call is to marry him.
— *Anonymous* [135]

If God had wanted us to make house calls, He would have given us better knees.
— *Anonymous* [135]

A doctor made a brief house call to one of his elderly patients. As he left the house, he told the patient's wife, "There's nothing wrong with your husband. He just thinks he's sick."

A few days later the doctor called his patient to see if his impression was correct.

"How is you husband today," he asked.

"He's worse," the woman said. "Now he thinks he's dead."

(See also Medical Practice, Primary Care)

~ HUMOR ~

He who laughs, lasts.
— *Mary Pettibone Poole* [250]

Everything is funny as long as it is happening to somebody else.
— *Will Rogers* [262]

If you see two doctors laughing, someone's in trouble.   — *Rip Pfeiffer, MD* [248]

Hilarity and good humor . . . help enormously both in the study and in the practice of medicine.   — *William Osler, MD* [27]

Wit happens.   — *Karyn Buxman, RN* [311]

The arrival of a good clown exercises a more beneficial influence upon the health of a town than twenty asses laden with drugs.   — *Thomas Sydenham* [180]

Humor is the good-natured side of a truth.   — *Mark Twain* [135]

Humor can be dissected, as a frog can, but the thing dies in the process and the innards are discouraging to any but the pure scientific mind.   — *E. B. White* [314]

A clown is like an aspirin, only he works twice as fast.   — *Groucho Marx* [180]

Wit is the sudden marriage of ideas which before their union were not perceived to have any relation.   — *Mark Twain* [12]

(See also Laughter)

~ HYPOCHONDRIACS ~

Hypochondria is the only disease I haven't got.   — *Anonymous* [217]

The best cure for hypochondria is to forget about your body and get interested in someone else's.   — *Goodman Ace* [322]

Hypochondria—The imaginary complaints of indestructible old ladies.   — *E. B. White* [315]

A motto for hypochondriacs:
There is no such thing as *just* a mole.
— *Fran Lebowitz* [(190)]

My husband does not let his good health get in the way of thinking that he could die at any minute.
— *Rita Rudner* [(271)]

Comment about a patient with years of imaginary bowel complaints:
When I die, it will not be my life which flashes before my eyes, but Mrs. P's bowel—all twenty feet of it. And it will not flash, but glide majestically, enabling me to examine it all in painful detail. And it will look entirely normal.
— *Keith Hopcraft, MD* [(162)]

Epitaph for a hypochondriac:
I told you I was sick!
— *Anonymous* [(186)]

What can you give the hypochondriac who has everything?
— A CAT Scan.

~ HYPOTHALAMUS ~

The hypothalamus is one of the most important parts of the human brain. In addition to other things, the hypothalamus controls the Four F's: fighting, fleeing, feeding, and reproduction.
— *Anonymous* [(135)]

(See also Brain)

I

~ ILLNESS ~

The great secret known to internists, but still hidden from the general public, is that most things get better by themselves. Most things, in fact, are better by morning.
— *Lewis Thomas, MD* [304]

Expectations are very low when you are sick. Basically, your time is spent on frequent naps and attending to your bodily functions, which is how we should live all the time.
— *Mark DePaolis, MD* [110]

How can I get sick? I've had everything already.
— *George Burns* [75]

It's a bad sign when the number of consultants on a case is greater than the number of members in the patient's family.
— *Rick Stevens, MD* [246]

If your time hasn't come, not even a doctor can kill you.
— *Meyer A. Perlstein, MD* [298]

I have gout, asthma, and seven other maladies, but am otherwise very well.
— *Sydney Smith* [298]

If you look like your passport photo, you're too ill to travel.
— *Will Kommen* [196]

One of the minor pleasures in life is to be slightly ill.
— *Harold Nicolson* [194]

I don't know which is harder, taking my body to the doctor or taking my car to the garage. I'm always afraid they'll find something I don't know about. The only advantage in taking my body to the doctor is that the doctor never asks me to leave it overnight.
— *Andy Rooney* [263]

I enjoy convalescence. It's the part that makes the illness worthwhile.

— *George Bernard Shaw* [279]

I used up all my sick days, so I'm calling in dead.

— *Anonymous* [135]

If you treat a sick child like an adult and a sick adult like a child, everything usually works out pretty well.

— *Ruth Carlisle* [322]

A woman accompanied her husband to the doctor. After the examination the doctor came out and said, "I don't like the way your husband looks."

"Neither do I," said the woman, "but he's good with the kids."

A doctor made a brief house call to one of his elderly patients. As he left the house, he told the patient's wife, "There's nothing wrong with your husband. He just thinks he's sick."

A few days later the doctor called his patient to see if his impression was correct.

"How is you husband today?" he asked.

"He's worse," the woman said. "Now he thinks he's dead."

My doctor likes to break things to me gently. The other day I asked him, "Doc, is it serious?" He said, "Only if you have plans for next year."

(See also Disease, Symptoms)

~ IMPOTENCE ~

I just took two Viagra; now I'm as hard as Chinese algebra.   — *Robin Williams* [135]

A hard man is good to find.

— *Mae West* [23]

What's the difference between anxiety and panic?

— Anxiety is the first time you can't do it a second time. Panic is the second time you can't do it the first time.

A man went to see a urologist because he was having a problem with impotence. After a thorough examination, the doctor told the man he had three options.

"The first treatment costs $5,000," the doctor said. "It consists of drug therapy supplemented with vitamins and minerals. This helps 25% of patients."

"The second treatment costs $10,000. It consists of physical therapy and weekly injections for six months. This approach works 50% of the time."

"The third treatment costs $20,000. It involves of reconstructive surgery, but has proven successful in over 90% of cases."

The doctor told the man to go home and discuss things with his wife.

The following week, the doctor met with the patient at a follow-up appointment.

"What did you decide?" the doctor asked.

"My wife decided to re-do the kitchen."

What do you give to the man who had everything?
— Viagra.

How is Viagra like Disneyland?
— You have to wait an hour for a three-minute ride.

(See also Penis, Sex)

~ INDIGESTION ~

To eat is human, to digest divine.   — *Charles T. Copeland* [(298)]

Dyspeptic: A man that can eat his cake and have it too.   — *Austin O'Malley* [(251)]

I would like to find a food that will give me heartburn immediately instead of at 3 o'clock in the morning.   — *John Barrymore* [(191)]

Daphne Moon: I'm making cheese puffs, pigs in a blanket, and tiny peanut butter sandwiches. Do you need anything else?
Dr. Frasier Crane: Yes, how about the number of the nearest gastroenterologist.
                          — *"Frasier"* [(131)]

My father was once rushed to the hospital from his hotel room with an apparent heart attack that, thank heavens, turned out to be an "acute gastric episode." That's the term hospitals use for five thousand dollars' worth of heartburn.

— *Christopher Buckley* (72)

Don't tell your friends about your indigestion. "How are you?" is a greeting, not a question.

— *Robert Benchley* (103)

Herbert Swope: What are you doing for dinner tonight?
George S. Kaufman: Digesting it. (116)

The fate of a nation has often depended upon the good or bad digestion of a prime minister.

— *Voltaire* (103)

(See also Gastrointestinal Tract)

~ INFECTIOUS DISEASE ~

There are only two things a child will share willingly—communicable diseases and his mother's age.

— *Benjamin Spock, MD* (293)

Infectious disease docs do it with culture and sensitivity.

— *Ludwig Lettau, MD* (246)

Little Miss Muffet sat on a tuffet
Eating a burger soufflé.
  Her mother then spied her,
  E Coli inside her,
An ambulance took her away.

— *John H. Hayes* (153)

Infectious Disease Definitions:
- Aerobe: A garment worn around the house.
- Antibody: No one in particular.
- Aseptic: One who doubts.
- Bullae: A tough guy.
- Fahrenheit: Very tall.
- Fester: Quicker.
- Influenzal: Having a lot of power.
- Lobar: A tavern for midgets.
- Node: Was aware of.

Bloopers & Malapropisms:
- A mother brought her 6-year-old to the office for a throat *sculpture*. (culture)
- The patient presented to the ICU with toxic *sock* syndrome. (shock)
- Dr. Weissman felt that it was a lymph node and we should sit on it.
- The urine culture grew greater than 10^5 staph *epididymis*. (epidermidis)
- The patient is a 4-year-old boy who has bacterial *conjunktivitis*. (conjunctivitis)
- The patient was dehydrated and had abnormal *electric lights*. (electrolytes)
- We will cover him with antibiotics for the next couple of days.
- The child has had vomiting and diarrhea for three days, so we recorded his *eyes and nose*. (I's & O's)
- The patient denies rigors or shaking chills, but her husband states that she was very hot in bed last night.
- The patient is a 63-year-old man with right upper *load* pneumonia. (lobe)

A young couple got married after an old-fashioned courtship that did not include any serious petting. When they arrived at their hotel room, the groom took the lead and began to get undressed. After he took off his shoes and socks, his bride looked at his feet and said, "What's wrong with your toes, they're all gnarled and twisted?"

"Oh, that," he said. "When I was a boy, I had a case of tolio."

"Don't you mean polio?" she asked.

"No," he answered. "It's like polio, but it involves your toes."

The man continued to get undressed and pretty soon took off his shirt and pants. His wife looked at his legs and said, "What happened to your knees, they're all scarred and swollen?"

"Oh, that," he said. "When I was a teenager, I had a case of kneasles."

"Don't you mean measles?" she asked.

"No," he answered. "It's like measles, but it involves your knees."

A few moments later, the man stood before his wife completely naked. She looked at her husband and said, " I see, you must have had a case of smallcox too."

A man walked into a doctor's office and the receptionist asked him why he was there.

"Shingles," the man answered.

So she took down his name, address, and insurance information and asked him to have a seat.

A few minutes later, a nursing assistant escorted the man to an examination room and asked him what he had.

"Shingles," the man answered.

So she recorded his vital signs and told him to wait.

Ten minutes later, a nurse came in and asked him what he had.

"Shingles," the man answered.

So she drew a routine blood count, did an EKG, and told him to take off all his clothes and wait for the doctor.

Twenty minutes later, the doctor came in and asked the man what he had.

"Shingles," the man answered.

The doctor said, "Where?"

The man said, "Out in my truck. I'm here to fix the roof."

Medical science has determined that one's attitude influences the susceptibility to illness, particularly infectious disease. Therefore, people who are cheerful and upbeat are less prone to illness than those who are pessimistic and malcontent. Thus, the surly bird gets the germ.

(See also Abscess, Antibiotics, Bacteria, Cephalosporins, Common Cold, Cough, Diarrhea, Fever, Hepatitis, Influenza, Lyme Disease, Mumps, Spinal Tap, Strep Throat, Venereal Disease, Vomiting, Zoonoses)

~ INFERTILITY ~

Sing a song of Clomid.
A pelvis full of dye;
Four and twenty studies
Your HMO won't buy.
When the tests are finished,
The docs and nurses sing,
"By the time we get you pregnant,
You won't own a thing."

— *Howard Bennett, MD* [47]

In vitro fertilization allows an egg and sperm cell to come together in the ideal environment, namely a glass specimen dish on a laboratory shelf.

— *Mark DePaolis, MD* [(108)]

Nowadays, women can have kids for other women through surrogate motherhood. Is that the ultimate favor or what? I think I'm a good friend. I'll help you move. Okay. But whatever comes out of me after nine months, I'm keeping. I don't care if it's a shoe.

— *Sue Kolinsky* [(96)]

Statements noted in medical records:
• Between you and me, we ought to be able to get this lady pregnant.
• Since she can't get pregnant with her husband, I thought you'd like to work her up.

Two college roommates, who hadn't seen each other in years, met for lunch at a trendy downtown restaurant. After catching up on things, the conversation turned to their husband's occupations.

"So what does George do for a living?" one of the women asked.

"He's an engineer," her friend answered. "What does Mark do?"

"He's an infertility specialist."

"That sounds like interesting work."

"Well," her friend said. "I'm the only wife I know who's thrilled every time her husband gets another woman pregnant."

An elderly man decided to get married again. The couple wanted to have a baby, but they had no luck so the man went to get his sperm count checked.

After doing a history and physical examination, the doctor handed the man a jar. "Take this home and bring a sample back in the morning."

The old man returned with an empty jar. "I tried," he said wearily. "I tried with my left hand. Nothing. I tried with my right hand. Nothing. I tried with both hands. Nothing. I asked my wife. She tried with both hands. Nothing. We even asked the lady across the street to try, but she couldn't do it either."

"You asked your neighbor?" the doctor said incredulously.

"Yes," the old man said. "None of us could get the lid off that jar."

(See also Artificial Insemination, Obstetrics)

~ INFLUENZA ~

I had the flu last week. I would have killed myself, but I was too weak to pick up the gun.
— *Rick Stevens, MD* [246]

~ INFORMED CONSENT ~

Why is it better to be a doctor than a patient? You're one of the few people who can actually give *Informed Consent* (not that you ever would).
— *Anne Eva Ricks, MD* [256]

Informed Consent, n. The only thing that stands between a surgeon and his 9-iron.
— *Howard Bennett, MD* [46]

A mistake from a medical center consent form:
It is very unlikely, though possible, that this treatment could result in your death. In previous studies, these side effects have been transient and have returned to normal after discontinuing the offending agent.   — *Anonymous* [214]

~ INJURIES ~

(See Accidents)

~ INNOVATIONS ~

If something is worth doing well, someone has probably already done it.
— *Leslie Bernstein, MD* [193]

~ INSANITY ~

Insanity is grounds for divorce in some states, grounds for marriage in all.
— *Tobias Smolett* [191]

Radar O'Reilly: Dr. Freedman, sometimes I talk to my teddy bear. Does that mean I'm crazy?
Dr. Freedman: Does he talk back to you?
Radar: Of course not.
Dr. Freedman: Then you're not crazy.   — *"M*A*S*H"* [200]

~ INSOMNIA ~

A recent study showed that if you're having trouble falling asleep, you should take two teaspoons of catnip in boiling water before going to bed. The only trouble is that instead of falling asleep in front of the TV, you fall asleep on top of the TV.   — *Jay Leno* [135]

Insomnia is a contagious disease transmitted from babies to parents.
— *Shannon Fife* [12]

A good cure for insomnia is to get plenty of sleep.   — *W. C. Fields* [217]

There once was a patient named Silya
Who asked, "Can insomnia kill ya?"
  "That depends," said her doc
  As he glanced at his clock,
"On whether you pay when I bill ya."   — *Howard Bennett, MD* [41]

Patient: Doctor, is it true that sleeping outdoors will cure insomnia?
Doctor: Yes. But sleeping indoors will do the same thing.

(See also Sleep)

~ INSURANCE ~

(See Health Insurance, Life Insurance)

~ INTENSIVE CARE ~

If I'm ever stuck on a respirator or a life support system, I definitely want to be unplugged—but not until I'm down to a size eight.   — *Henriette Mantel* [96]

Principles of Intensive Care:
• Air goes in and out.
• Blood goes 'round and 'round.
• Oxygen is good.   — *Robert Matz, MD* [202]

How many intensivists does it take to change a light bulb?
—None. The bulb has a DNR order on the chart.

(See also Emergency Medicine)

~ INTERNAL MEDICINE ~

An internist is someone who knows everything and does nothing. A surgeon is someone who knows nothing and does everything. A pathologist is someone who knows everything and does everything but too late.   — *Anonymous* [94]

The difference between an internist and a pediatrician is how you feel when your patient pees on you.   — *Andy Biles* [135]

Surgeons do it. Internists talk about it. Radiologists just like to look at the pictures.   — *Anonymous* [94]

Loeb's Laws of Medicine:
• If what you're doing is working, keep doing it.
• If what you're doing is not working, stop doing it.
• If you don't know what to do, don't do anything.
• Above all, never let a surgeon get your patient. [201]

As a member of the American Board of Internal Medicine, I tried for six years, unsuccessfully, to get a clinical practice question into the exam to which the correct answer was "nothing." — *Alvan Feinstein, MD* [126]

A surgeon, an internist, and a family practitioner go duck hunting.

The surgeon sees a duck, shouts, "Duck!" and shoots it down.

The internist sees a duck, shouts, "Duck! Rule out quail! Rule out pheasant!" and shoots it down.

The family practitioner sees a duck and blasts it out of the sky with a burst of machine-gun fire. As the tattered carcass falls to the ground, he remarks, "I don't know what the hell it was, but I sure got it."

(For a variation on this joke, see page 197.)

How can you tell the difference between an internist and an orthopedist when they're rushing to get on an elevator?
— The internist holds the door open with his hands; the orthopod uses his head.

Mark went to his internist for his annual checkup. After a thorough examination, the doctor said, "I've got some good news and some bad news."

"What's the good news?" the patient asked.

"The good news is that my son just got into Harvard Medical School."

"And the bad news?"

"You're paying for it."

How many internists does it take to change a light bulb?
— I don't know. Let me check a reference on that and I'll get back to you.

(See also Medical Practice, Physical Diagnosis, Primary Care, VA Hospitals)

~ INTERNSHIP & RESIDENCY ~

Don't get sick in July. — *Anonymous* [94]

To err is human, to sleep divine. — *Residency Slogan* [94]

Every ward has a silver lining.

— *Howard Bennett, MD* [48]

The main difference between medical school and residency is that with one you pay to become sleep deprived and with the other, someone pays you.

— *Howard Bennett, MD* [43]

House Officer's Comment:
If I've done anything to be sorry for, I'm willing to be forgiven.

— *Anonymous* [203]

On ward rounds:
Be wary of medical students who follow you into the bathroom.

— *Anonymous* [135]

The quickest way to guarantee an admission to the ICU is to tell someone you're having an easy night on-call.

— *Anonymous* [135]

There are three goals that all residents aspire to:
• To be really good at procedures.
• To out diagnose their attendings.
• To fall asleep at Grand Rounds without drooling.

— *Ryan James, MD* [246]

Comparing residency training to medical school is like comparing a blown pupil to anisocoria.

— *Howard Bennett, MD* [35]

Rules of the Ward:
• Your sickest patient never speaks English.
• There are no interesting cases after midnight.
• Never pull a good IV.
• There is no such thing as too much tape.
• Old charts are always missing.
• There's always more scut to do.
• Never trip on your way to a code.
• The best vein is always the last one you check.
• Never use small words when big ones will do.
• When all else fails, turf the patient.

How many residents does it take to change a light bulb?
— Four. The first three refuse to do it because it isn't their bulb. The fourth says he'll do it, but complains that he has ten other bulbs to change first.

(See also Attendings, Chief Resident, Education, Roundsmanship, VA Hospitals)

~ IRON DEFICIENCY ~

Are you aware that women require twice as much iron as men? Very few of them are getting it, and for this reason they suffer from sluggishness, mid-afternoon fatigue, and an inability to put up with small children.   — *Russell Baker* [21]

(See also Hematology)

~ ITCHING ~

'Tis better than riches
To scratch when it itches.   — *Anonymous* [298]

The severity of an itch is inversely proportional to its location.
                                                                                        — *Anonymous* [135]

One bliss for which there is no match
Is when you itch, to up and scratch.   — *Ogden Nash* [228]

(See also Dermatology)

~ IVs ~

Never pull a good IV.   — *Anonymous* [94]

The best vein is always the last one you check.   — *Anonymous* [94]

There is no such thing as too much tape.

— *Anonymous* [94]

There are two kinds of adhesive tape—that which won't stay on and that which won't come off.

— *Maria Telesco* [302]

(See also Blood & Blood Drawing)

J

~ JARGON ~

I am tired of people saying that doctors can't speak English. This is just not true. Many of them know how to speak English perfectly well, they simply choose not to.   — *Mark DePaolis, MD* [109]

Never use a big word when a bigger one will do.   — *Howard Bennett, MD* [48]

I know there are professors in this country who "ligate" arteries. Other surgeons only "tie" them, and it stops the bleeding just as well.
— *Oliver Wendell Holmes, Sr., MD* [298]

When there's no explanation they give it a name, which, of course, immediately explains everything.   — *Martin H. Fischer* [103]

Ad-i-ad-o-cho-kin-e-sis
Is a term that will bolster my thesis,
    That 'tis idle to seek
    Such precision in Greek,
When confusion it only increases.   — *Horace B. and Ava C. English* [121]

It's one of those hospitals where they have code words for unpleasant things. For instance, patients never die, they just take a turn for the hearse.
— *Anonymous* [234]

~ JOGGING ~

The only reason I would take up jogging is so I could hear heavy breathing again.   — *Erma Bombeck* [96]

The first time I see a jogger smiling, I'll consider it. — *Joan Rivers* [135]

A friend of mine runs marathons. He always talks about this "runner's high," but he has to go twenty-six miles for it. That's why I smoke and drink. I get the same feeling from a flight of stairs. — *Larry Miller* [96]

I don't jog. If I die, I want to be sick. — *Abe Lemons* [196]

I belong to Athletes Anonymous. When I get the urge to jog, I call up two friends. They rush right over with a six-pack and talk me out of it.

— *Will Durst* [117]

(See also Exercise)

$\mathcal{K}$

~ KIDNEYS ~

There was a young fellow named Sydney,
Who drank till he ruined his kidney.
   It shriveled and shrank,
   As he sat there and drank,
But he had lots of fun doin' it didney?
— Don Marquis [85]

The only indication for a kidney biopsy is having two kidneys.
— Anonymous [94]

(See also Nephrology)

~ KNEES ~

If God had intended man to engage in strenuous sports, He would have given us better knees.
— Robert Ray [62]

Two weeks ago I took care of a lady who had fallen. After I examined her swollen knee, I told her to go home, elevate it, and put ice on it. Twenty minutes later she called me on the phone: "I talked to Mabel, my maid, who thinks we ought to put heat on this knee." I told her, "You know, this morning at breakfast I was talking to my maid, Ruthie, and she said to put ice on it."
— Christian Ramsey, Jr, MD [252]

(See also Arthritis, Orthopedics)

~ KREBS CYCLE ~

A doctor doesn't need to know the Krebs Cycle, but at least he should have forgotten it.

— *Anonymous* [135]

The Krebs Cycle is a series of complicated biochemical reactions that show how everything we eat turns to fat.

— *Howard Bennett, MD* [48]

$\mathcal{L}$

~ LAB TESTS ~

If you order a lab test to reassure a patient, the results will always be abnormal.
— Howard Bennett, MD [48]

The lab knows me so well, they call ahead to tell me they've lost my patient's specimen.
— Ryan James, MD [246]

A little stool, a little pus,
Blood and guts don't bother us.
— Sign in a medical lab [135]

Bennett's Axiom on Lab Results:
• Unexpected lab results will not correct themselves no matter how many times you look at the chart.
• Corollary No. 1: Unexpected lab results will not correct themselves no matter how long you keep the patient's chart on your desk. [48]

(See also Blood & Blood Drawing, Diagnosis)

~ LAST WORDS (REAL AND SUGGESTED) ~

Big deal! I'm used to dust.
— Erma Bombeck [184]

I'm dying, but otherwise I'm in very good health.
— Edith Sitwell [62]

In case my life should end with the cannibals, I hope they will write on my tombstone, "We have eaten Dr. Schweitzer. He was good to the end."
— Albert Schweitzer, MD [268]

Excuse My Dust.   — *Dorothy Parker* [238]

I'm dying from the help of too many physicians.   — *Alexander the Great* [298]

All things considered, I'd rather be in Philadelphia.   — *W. C. Fields* [268]

I told you I was ill.   — *Spike Milligan* [197]

Die, my dear doctor! That's the last thing I'll do.   — *Lord Palmerston* [103]

On the bedroom curtains in the room where he was dying:
Either they go or I do.   — *Oscar Wilde (Attrib.)* [283]

(See also Death)

~ LAUGHTER ~

Laughter is the shortest distance between two people.   — *Victor Borge* [180]

Laughter is a form of internal jogging. It moves your organs around. It enhances respiration. It is an igniter of great expectations.   — *Norman Cousins* [261]

Laughter and tears are both responses to frustration and exhaustion . . . I myself prefer to laugh, since there is less cleaning up to do afterward.
                                                         — *Kurt Vonnegut* [180]

You don't stop laughing because you grow old; you grow old because you stop laughing.   — *Michael Pritchard* [105]

Life does not cease to be funny when people die any more than it ceases to be serious when people laugh.   — *George Bernard Shaw* [320]

(See also Humor)

~ Lawyers ~

Feed a cold, starve a lawyer.

— Oscar London, MD [192]

It's unfair to believe everything we hear about lawyers . . . some of it might not be true.

— Gerald F. Lieberman [191]

A CAT scan a day keeps the lawyers away.

— Howard Bennett, MD [40]

While not as popular as they once were, people still like doctors better than lawyers . . . Even a doctor who writes columns about space alien abductions and cartoon characters could theoretically help you if he happened to find you on the side of the road after an accident, whereas most lawyers would just sue you for obstructing traffic and wrongful bleeding. *— Mark DePaolis, MD* [108]

I tried to get out of jury duty last week, but it didn't work. When I told the judge that lawyers give me hives, he showed me his bottle of Benadryl and told me to deal with it like everyone else. *— Howard Bennett, MD* [48]

Cardiologists believe that experiments in dogs are essential, but antivivisectionists oppose animal research. There is a solution to this dilemma—use lawyers instead of dogs. The one problem, of course, is extrapolating the results from lawyers to humans. *— Charles Hennekens, MD* [155]

Even though I'm a doctor, I have the same interests as regular folks. When I go to a restaurant I say to myself, "What's the ambience? How good is the food? Do they let lawyers eat here?" *— Molly Ryan, MD* [246]

The brain uses less power than a 100-watt bulb. With lawyers, it's much less.

— Anonymous [135]

Why have laboratories switched from rats to lawyers in their experiments?
• There's no shortage of lawyers.
• You don't get attached to them.
• There are some things even rats won't do.

A man was standing in line at a movie theater when suddenly he felt someone massaging his shoulders. He turned around to the woman behind him and said, "Hey lady, what do you think you're doing?"

"Oh, I'm sorry," she said. "You see, I'm a chiropractor and I could see that you were all tensed up and so, without thinking, I started to rub your shoulders to release the tension and make you relax. I really apologize."

"Well, you ought to apologize," he blustered. "You shouldn't be taking your job out of the office. I'm a lawyer. Do you see me screwing the guy in front of me?"

Julie McCoy went to see her gynecologist for a routine checkup before her fourth marriage. After the examination the doctor said, "I'm sorry if I look a little confused, but I noticed that you're still a virgin, and I was wondering how that's possible?"

"Well," Ms. McCoy said, "my first husband was an internist and all he did was talk about it. My second husband was a psychiatrist and all he did was analyze it. My third husband was a surgeon and he was never around to do anything about it. But now I'm marrying a lawyer, so I know I'll get screwed."

A doctor finally got to his table after breaking away from a patient who sought his advice for a medical problem.

"Do you think I should send her a bill?" the doctor asked a lawyer who was sitting next to him.

"Why not?" the lawyer said. "You rendered professional services by giving advice."

"Thanks," the doctor said. "I think I'll do just that."

When the doctor went to his office the following day, he found a note from the lawyer. It read, "For legal services, $50."

From a courtroom transcript:
Q: Doctor, did you check for a pulse before you performed the autopsy?
A: No.
Q: Did you check the blood pressure?
A: No.
Q: So then, it is possible that the patient was still alive when you began the autopsy?
A: No.
Q: How can you be sure, Doctor?
A: Because his brain was sitting on my desk in a jar.
Q: But could the patient have still been alive nonetheless?
A: Only if he was a lawyer.

A doctor, an engineer, and a lawyer stood outside the pearly gates, awaiting their admittance to heaven. St. Peter suddenly appeared and announced he could only admit one—the person with the oldest profession.

"That's me," the doctor said confidently. "As soon as God created Adam, he performed an operation. He took a rib from Adam's side and created Eve. Surgery is the oldest profession."

"Wait a minute," replied the engineer. "Before God created Adam and Eve, he overcame the chaos that existed and constructed the earth in six days. Engineering came before surgery."

"You're both wrong," said the lawyer. "Who do you think created the chaos?"

How many lawyers does it take to change a light bulb?
— How many can you afford?

(See also Malpractice)

~ LECTURES ~

When lecturing, never use a simple sentence when a complex one will do.
— *Ian Rose, MD* [266]

The likelihood of staying awake at a lecture is inversely related to the number of slides.
— *Roger P. Smith, MD* [290]

A lecture is an occasion when you numb one end to benefit the other.
— *John Gould* [168]

If there is anyone in the back who doesn't hear me, please don't raise your hand because I am also nearsighted.
— *W. H. Auden* [103]

Superfluity of lecturing causes ischial bursitis.
— *William Osler, MD* [27]

Any student will tell you that the longest five minutes in the world are the last five minutes of a lecture, while the shortest five minutes are the last five minutes of an exam.
— *Karl Newell* [217]

The lecture method of instruction is based on the idea that the instructor's notebook can be transferred directly to the student's notebook without passing through the brain of either. — *Darrell Huff* [268]

When audiences come to see authors lecture, it is in the hope that we'll be funnier to look at than to read. — *Sinclair Lewis* [124]

A psychology professor was annoyed by a student who was always knitting during his lectures. One day he stopped in mid-sentence and said to the student, "Young woman, do you know what you are really doing when you knit like that? You're masturbating."

"Well, professor," replied the student, "I'll do it my way and you do it yours."

How many lecturers does it take to change a light bulb?
— None. The instructions are all in the handout.

(See also Academia, Continuing Medical Education, Education)

~ LIFE ~

Two leading Congressional scientists, Senator Helms and Representative Hyde, have been doing pioneering research on the nature of life. This has produced the Helms-Hyde theory which states that scientific fact can be established by a majority vote of the United States Congress. — *Russel Baker* [21]

Coach: How's life Norm?
Norm Peterson: It's a dog-eat-dog world, and I'm wearing Milkbone underwear. — *"Cheers"* [87]

Life is what happens to you while you are making other plans. — *Robert Balzer* [111]

On the definition of life:
Life is anything that dies when you stomp on it. — *Dave Barry* [24]

Life is a sexually transmitted disease.   — *Guy Bellamy* [12]

There's an old joke. Two elderly women are at a Catskills resort and one of 'em says, "Boy, the food at this place is really terrible." The other one says, "Yeah, I know, and such small portions." Well, that's essentially how I feel about life. Full of loneliness and misery and suffering . . . and it's all over much too soon.
                              — *Woody Allen & Marshall Brickman* [9]

If I had to live my life again I'd make all the same mistakes—only sooner.
                                          — *Tallulah Bankhead* [195]

Don't take your life too seriously—you'll never get out of it alive.
                                            — *Elbert Hubbard* [268]

~ LIFE INSURANCE ~

On insurance physicals:
I have done many of these physicals on other people; and as far as I can tell, an insurance physical can only determine one thing—whether or not you are going to die during the physical.   — *Mark DePaolis, MD* [108]

(See also Health Insurance)

~ LIPOSUCTION ~

A lot of our current medical practices will seem ridiculous years from now. Actually, some of them are pretty silly even today. For example, when Hippocrates said, "First, do no harm," he could never in his wildest dreams have imagined anything like liposuction.   — *Mark DePaolis, MD* [108]

They've got these new techniques where they can suck the fat out of one part of your body and put it into other parts. Boy, that's a bad idea. I want them to suck the fat out of my body and put it into Cindy Crawford.   — *Rita Rudner* [135]

Liposuction sounded good, till I read they can accidentally suck out internal organs that you're still using. — *Rita Rudner* [135]

(See also Obesity, Plastic Surgery)

~ LIVER ~

Liver, n. A large red organ thoughtfully provided by nature to be bilious with. — *Ambrose Bierce* [298]

(See also Hepatitis)

~ LONGEVITY ~

The secret of a long life is to stay busy, get plenty of exercise, and don't drink too much. Then again, don't drink too little. — *Herman Smith-Johannsen, at 103* [12]

If I'd known I was gonna live this long, I'd have taken better care of myself. — *Eubie Blake, at 100* [55]

On the secret of life:
Swim, dance a little, go to Paris every August, and live within walking distance of two hospitals. — *Horatio Luro, at 80* [62]

Sophie Tucker's response, at age 80, when asked the secret of her longevity:
Keep breathing. [103]

(See also Death, Life)

~ LUNGS ~

A medical chest specialist is long-winded about the short-winded. — *Kenneth T. Bird, MD* [298]

Apnea, n. Form of greeting to one whose arrival has been unduly delayed; as "We was wondering what apnea." — *H. S. Grannatt* [144]

A woman went to see a new doctor who turned out to be very handsome. He put his hand on her back and asked her to say "Ninety-nine."

"Ninety-nine," she said.

"Good," he said. "Now I'm going to put my hand on your throat, and I want you to say Ninety-nine again."

"Ninety-niiiiine," she purred.

"Fine," he said. "Now I'm going to put my hand on your chest, and I want you to say 'Ninety-nine' one last time."

"Okay," she said. "One, two, three, four . . ."

(See also Asthma, Cough, Diaphragm, Radiology, Smoking)

~ LYME DISEASE ~

On how to avoid tick bites when camping:
It's useful to hike with a partner so you can check each other over, both clothed and—at least twice a day—unclothed, giving special attention to patches of hair. This procedure is not recommended for a first date. — *Paul McHugh* [208]

A columnist's response to the above quote:
I can hear the guy whining now—"OK, don't take your clothes off. Get Lyme disease. See if I care." — *Herb Caen* [79]

M

~ MALPRACTICE ~

Malpractice, n. According to your current doctor, medicine as practiced by all of your physicians before him. — *George Thomas, MD & Lee Schreiner, MD* [303]

When I first started out in practice, I would lie awake at night worrying about my patients. Now I lie awake worrying about their lawyers. — *Howard Fischer, MD* [246]

Doctor: What do you want to be when you grow up?
Child: A doctor.
Doctor: What's the most important thing to remember to be a good doctor?
Child: Don't get sued. — *Interview with a 5-year-old* [135]

A malpractice lawyer, an HMO administrator, and a Medicare auditor jump off the Empire State Building at the same time. Which one hits the ground first?
— Who cares?

A lawyer was attempting to lighten his cross-examination of an anesthesiologist who was a plaintiff in a malpractice case.
   "I guess that means you and I are in the same business because we both put people to sleep," the lawyer joked.
   "Yes," replied the doctor, "but I wake them up."

(See also Lawyers)

~ MAMMOGRAMS ~

You never realize how long a minute is until you get a mammogram.
— *Jan Henkelman* [246]

Many women are needlessly afraid of mammograms. By taking a few minutes every day to do the following exercise, you will be totally prepared for the study:
• Freeze two metal bookends overnight.
• Strip to waist.
• Invite a stranger into the room.
• Place one bookend on each side of your breast.
• Press the bookends together as hard as you can.
• Hold that position for five seconds.
• Don't breathe.
• Repeat with the other breast.
• Make an appointment with the stranger to repeat the procedure next year.

(See also Breast Exams)

~ MANAGED CARE ~

Changing HMOs is like changing rooms on the Titanic. *— Anonymous* [135]

I called one of my friends the other day to see if he wanted to go to a ballgame with me. He told me he'd love to, but he recently changed jobs and I was no longer on his list of preferred friends. *— Howard Bennett, MD* [48]

Asking a primary care doc what he thinks about HMO administrators is like asking a litter box what it thinks about cats. *— Ryan James, MD* [246]

I live in an area with a lot of children so my teenage daughter is in high demand as a babysitter. We just put her on a capitated basis and she covers about 50 "child lives" in our neighborhood. So now when parents call, she tries to convince them to rent a movie instead. *— Stu Silverstein, MD* [246]

My kids love to play doctor. Just last week, my 6-year-old examined one of his friends who had a stomachache. Ryan told Peter he needed a CAT scan, but Peter's big sister said their HMO wouldn't approve it without a second opinion. Ryan said he'd been a specialist for a zillion years and he'd be damned if some insurance company would question his clinical judgment. He said if Peter couldn't get the scan he wasn't playing anymore. So he came home and took a nap. *— Howard Bennett, MD* [48]

If there was any justice in this world, HMO executives would always be in the placebo group.
                                                                                                                         — *Anonymous* [135]

Mary had a little lump
That soon began to grow.
And every one that Mary saw
Said, "Boy, that lump should go."
She went to see her doc one day
To get the lump removed.
But since it was cosmetic,
It couldn't be approved.
                                                                                                         — *Howard Bennett, MD* [45]

The CEO of a managed care company dies and goes to heaven, where he meets St. Peter at the Pearly Gates.

"I want to be admitted to heaven," the CEO demands. "I've lived a good life, and I've made health care more affordable."

"You can come in," St. Peter answers, "but you're only authorized for two days."

Managed Care Questions & Answers:
Q: Can I get coverage for preexisting conditions?
A: Certainly. As long as they don't require any treatment.
Q: Do all diagnostic procedures require pre-certification?
A: No. Only those you need.
Q: How difficult will it be to choose the doctor I want?
A: It's as easy as choosing your parents.
Q: What happens if I want to try alternative forms of medicine?
A: You'll need to find alternative forms of payment.

A malpractice lawyer, an HMO administrator, and a Medicare auditor jump off the Empire State Building at the same time. Which one hits the ground first?
— Who cares?

What are the top five reasons to work for an HMO?
• You get a free tote bag with the plan's logo on it.
• It gives you something to brag about at college reunions.
• It's a challenge to manage patients without any lab work.
• Your accountant thinks you should be in a lower tax bracket.
• Lawyers rarely belong to HMOs.

How many managed care reviewers does it take to change a light bulb?
— Five.
• The first receives the authorization forms and puts them at the bottom of the pile.
• The second puts the pile in a storage closet.
• The third refuses to authorize the light bulb change because the forms were never processed.
• The fourth processes the resubmitted authorization forms.
• The fifth authorizes a 40-watt bulb because a lower wattage bulb uses less electricity.

A doctor was having breakfast at a diner when he looked at the snow piling up in the street. "Think the roads are clear enough to go to work?" he mused.

The waiter shrugged his shoulders and said, "I guess that depends on whether you work for an HMO or not."

What are five rejected names for managed care companies?
• McHealth Care
• Suboptimum Choice
• Equivocare
• Premiums Plus
• You'll Get That Procedure Over Our Dead Body Health Plan

(See also Health Insurance)

~ MARRIAGE ~

Keep your eyes wide open before marriage, half shut afterward.
— Benjamin Franklin [169]

Married men live longer than single men. But married men are a lot more willing to die.
— Johnny Carson [307]

I've been married fourteen years and I have three kids. Obviously, I breed well in captivity.
— Roseanne Barr [197]

Marriage isn't a word . . . it's a sentence.   — *Anonymous* [217]

Marriage is a wonderful institution, but who wants to live in an institution?
                                                              — *Groucho Marx* [12]

To keep your marriage brimming
With love in the marriage cup,
Whenever you're wrong, admit it;
Whenever you're right, shut up.   — *Ogden Nash* [217]

Marriage confers one very special privilege—only a married person can get
divorced.   — *Ashleigh Brilliant* [66]

Luna Schlosser: You haven't had sex in 200 years?
Miles Monroe: Two hundred and four—if you count my marriage.
                                                      — *Woody Allen, "Sleeper"* [5]

Before marriage, a man will lie awake all night thinking about something you
said; after marriage, he'll fall asleep before you finish saying it.
                                                            — *Helen Rowland* [12]

Before accepting a marriage proposal, take a good look at his father. If he's still
handsome, witty, and has all his teeth . . . marry him instead.   — *Diane Jordan* [311]

We sleep in separate rooms, we have dinner apart, we take separate vacations—
we're doing everything we can to keep our marriage together.
                                                        — *Rodney Dangerfield* [12]

I don't think I'll get married again. I'll just find a woman I don't like and give
her a house.   — *Lewis Grizzard* [148]

Bigamy is having one husband too many. Monogamy is the same.
                                                              — *Anonymous* [195]

They say the secret to a successful marriage is just don't go to bed angry. So I
stayed awake for two years.   — *Wendy Liebman* [135]

Marrying a man is like buying something you've been admiring for a long time in a shop window. You may love it when you get it home, but it doesn't always go with everything else in the house.   — *Jean Kerr* [174]

Clerk: You know what the fastest way to a man's heart is?
Roseanne: Yeah, through his chest.   — *"Roseanne"* [267]

Married people don't have to exercise because our attitude is "They've seen us naked already—and they like it."   — *Carol Montgomery* [67]

Any woman who still thinks marriage is a fifty-fifty proposition is only proving that she doesn't understand either men or percentages.
                  — *Florence Kennedy* [310]

A woman accompanied her husband to the doctor. After the examination the doctor came out and said, "I don't like the way your husband looks."
   "Neither do I," said the woman, "but he's good with the kids."

A psychologist told a colleague, "Half of my patients come to me because they're married and the other half because they're not."

A middle-aged man was walking along the beach one day when he ran into an old lamp that was buried in the sand. He picked up the lamp and rubbed off the sand when all of a sudden a genie appeared.
   "Your wish is my command," the genie said.
   "Are you really a genie?" the man asked.
   "Yes," the genie said, "but I'm tired of this gig so get on with your lousy wish already."
   "Well," the man said, "I've always wanted to go to Hawaii, but I'm afraid to fly. I want you to build a bridge that goes all the way from San Francisco to Hawaii."
   "Are you crazy?" the genie said. "I'm too old and tired to do that. Pick something else."
   "Okay," the man said. "My wife and I have been married for twenty years, but she's never really understood me. I want you to fix it so she'll appreciate me more."
   "Alright," the genie said. "Do you want four lanes on that bridge or six?"

"It was just awful," the man told his psychiatrist. "I was in San Francisco on business, and I wired my wife that I'd be back a day early. I rushed home from the airport and found her in bed with my best friend. I don't get it. How could she do this to me?"

"Well," said the psychiatrist after a long pause, "maybe she didn't get your telegram."

(See also Divorce, Sex)

~ Masturbation ~

If God had intended us not to masturbate, he would have made our arms shorter.
— *George Carlin* [67]

We have reason to believe that man first walked upright to free his hands for masturbation.
— *Lily Tomlin* [135]

Don't knock masturbation—it's sex with someone I love.
— *Woody Allen* [9]

Surgeon General Jocelyn Elders resigned because of opposition to her plans to make masturbation a high school course. Damn, just when there's something I can finally teach.
— *Robin Williams* [67]

Masturbation is nothing to be ashamed of; it's nothing to be particularly proud of either.
— *Matt Groening* [150]

A psychology professor was annoyed by a student who was always knitting during his lectures. One day he stopped in mid-sentence and said to the student, "Young woman, do you know what you are really doing when you knit like that? You're masturbating."

"Well, professor," replied the student, "I'll do it my way and you do it yours."

An elderly woman was making dinner one night when in comes her 13-year-old grandson. "So, Sidney, what did you learn in school today?"

"We had sex education today, grandma."

"Sex education. What's that?"

"We learn about things like erections and vaginas and—"

She cuts him off, "Stop, I don't ever want to hear that kind of language coming out of you! Now go up to your room. You'll get no dinner tonight!"

Thirty minutes later the boy's mother comes home and asks where Sidney is.

"I sent him to his room," the old woman answers. "I asked him what he learned in school today. He said 'sex education' and then began using the filthiest words I ever heard. I can't even repeat them."

"Mom, that's what they teach kids these days. You asked him a question and he gave you an honest answer."

The grandmother felt bad now, so she goes upstairs to apologize to her grandson and ask him to come down to dinner. When she opens the door, she finds him in the corner masturbating.

"Sidney," she says, "when you're done with your homework . . ."

(See also Penis, Sex)

~ MEDIA ~

If you're unencumbered with the facts, you can say anything you want.
— *E. R. McFadden, MD* [207]

I'm getting tired of being in the dark about the latest medical advances. I guess it's my own fault. All I ever read are textbooks and medical journals . . . What I should be reading are the publications sold at supermarket checkout counters, like the *National Enquirer*. How else would I know that it is now possible to reverse the natural aging process, or that people can now perform their own liver transplants in the privacy of their own homes. — *Mark DePaolis, MD* [108]

(See also TV Doctors)

~ MEDICAL EDUCATION ~

(See Education)

~ MEDICAL LITERATURE ~

If you quote an article that you haven't read, someone will always ask for the reference. *— Anonymous* [94]

The trouble with facts is that there are so many of them.
— Samuel McChord Crothers [217]

Never consult a textbook that is older than the youngest medical student on your service. *— Howard Fischer, MD* [210]

If you look something up in a two volume text, the information you need will always be in the volume you didn't pick. *— Molly Ryan, MD* [246]

I file articles like a child eating spinach—there are new piles every few minutes, but nothing disappears. *— Howard Bennett, MD* [43]

The trouble with quoting the literature is that someone might actually be listening.
— Anonymous [135]

What do jokes and medical articles have in common?
a. They both get misquoted a lot.
b. Everybody wants to write one.
c. You can never remember one when you need to.
d. All of the above.

(See also Continuing Medical Education)

~ MEDICAL PRACTICE ~

There are two types of services in our society—those that require appointments and those where you wait in line. Then there are doctor's visits, where you get to do both. *— Howard Bennett, MD* [40]

We make money the old fashioned way: we double-book for it.

— *Ryan James, MD* [246]

A friend of mine has a solo practice in San Francisco. Last year he sold shares in the practice and went public. At the first stockholder's meeting, they voted to never let him take vacation.

— *Larry Bauer, MD* [246]

Telephones and eggs Benedict are the leading causes of premature death among doctors.

— *Oscar London, MD* [192]

Dr. Wicksteed: The longer I practice medicine, the more convinced I am that there are only two types of cases—those that involve taking the trousers off and those that don't.

— *Alan Bennett, "Habeas Corpus"* [31]

Medical Equivalents to "The Check is in the Mail":
• I can be at your office in 10 minutes.
• I'm faxing you that report right now.
• Your test results should be back tomorrow.
• The doctor will call you right back.
• I'm sure your insurance will cover this.
• The doctor is only slightly behind.

— *Larry Kravitz, MD* [210]

Your diploma only starts you in practice; it's your diplomacy that keeps you there.

— *Philip A. Kilbourne, MD* [176]

If you think you're indispensable, check your appointment book a week after you drop dead.

— *Oscar London, MD* [192]

(See also Advice, Art of Medicine, Computers, Experience, House Calls, Night Call, Paperwork, Patients & Patient Care, Retirement, Treatment, Waiting Room)

~ Medical Records ~

Scientists estimate that medical student notes account for more than 60% of a chart's weight.   — *Frederick L. Brancati, MD* [64]

When in doubt, write illegibly.   — *Howard Bennett, MD* [40]

How can you hide a $100 bill from a surgeon?
— Put it in a medical record.

~ Medical School ~

Starting third year is like going to a foreign country. You don't speak the language, you don't understand the customs, and the natives are not necessarily friendly.   — *Anne Eva Ricks, MD* [255]

Training for the Olympics is a lot like going to medical school—before you realize what you've gotten yourself into, it's too late to get out.
                                    — *Alan Mouchawar, MD* [225]

The general practitioner's association with the bowels begins with the digestion of large amounts of information in medical school. Quite often this intellectual nutrition is in a high fiber form; much of it is unabsorbed and goes straight through.   — *J. Dowden, MD* [115]

Masochists have an interesting array of choices for the expression of their symptomatology. Some choose alcoholism; some choose drug dependence; some choose excessive risk taking, or even going to medical school.
                                    — *Charles Morgan, MD* [224]

To most people, medical school means dissecting dead bodies and memorizing the names of all 203 bones, in between required classes on golf and bad penmanship. This is just not true. Bad penmanship is an elective.
                                    — *Mark DePaolis, MD* [108]

The main difference between medical school and residency is that with one you pay to become sleep deprived and with the other, someone pays you.

— *Howard Bennett, MD* [43]

Rules of the Wards:
• Remain conscious at all times.
• Avoid maligning the field in which you are rotating.
• Be ready for the $64,000 question—What are you going into?

— *Anne Eva Ricks, MD* [255]

When the team captain on medicine says to the third year student, "Do we have an EKG on Mr. Morris?" what he really means is, "Go do an EKG on Mr. Morris, interpret it, and bring it back to me—before attending rounds."

— *Anne Eva Ricks, MD* [256]

A patient went to the doctor for his annual checkup. After a thorough examination, the doctor said, "I've got some good news and some bad news."

"What's the good news?" the patient said.

"My son just got into Harvard Medical School."

"And the bad news?"

"You're paying for it."

(See also Anatomy, Education, Lectures)

~ MEDICAL STUDENTS ~

O'Leary's Law: Give medical students a 50/50 chance of reaching the correct answer and they will almost always be wrong. [216]

A medical student is someone who knows less than anyone else around him, inanimate objects not included.

— *Howard Bennett, MD* [32]

Motto for 4th year med students:
Eat when you can; sleep when you can; make yourself scarce.

— *Caren Glassman, MD* [246]

As a medical student, I remember following my interns wherever they went. If my intern went to the nursing station, I went to the nursing station. If my intern went to the bedside, I went to the bedside. If my intern went to the bathroom, I went to the bathroom. Sometimes my interns thought I was too enthusiastic—especially the women.

— Ryan James, MD [246]

The most important thing medical students need to consider when picking a specialty is which bodily fluid is least offensive to them. *— Howard Bennett, MD* [33]

Once I trusted a student to write life and death orders for ventilator settings and dopamine drips in the ICU, but he failed me—he was sent to get Moo Shu Pork for the team and he *forgot the plum sauce*. Clearly, he was a failure as a medical student. *— Anne Eva Ricks, MD* [757]

Scissors, n. An instrument used by medical students to cut surgical knots too short or too long. *— Howard Bennett, MD* [46]

If the radiology resident and the BMS (Best Medical Student) both see a lesion on the chest x-ray, there can be no lesion there. *— Samuel Shem, MD* [281]

There are two types of people who work in hospitals—those who think medical students are a pain in the butt and those who want to date them.

— Howard Bennett, MD [48]

There are two rules that all medical students must learn:
• Rule #1. The attending is always right.
• Rule #2. Don't forget Rule #1. *— Howard Bennett, MD* [40]

Show me a BMS (Best Medical Student) who only triples my work and I will kiss his feet. *— Samuel Shem, MD* [281]

The attending physician put a patient's x-ray on the view box and turned to the medical student beside him.

"As you can see, one of the patient's legs is two inches shorter than the other because of a deformed tibia. This causes the patient to limp. Now, what would you do in a case like this?"

"Well, doctor," the student said. "I guess I'd limp too."

A medical student was taking a history during his course in physical diagnosis.

"Did your father die a natural death?" the student inquired.

"Oh, no," the patient said. "He had a doctor."

How many medical students does it take to change a light bulb?

— Three. One to hold the bulb, one to read the manual, and one to call the attending when it won't come out.

How many attendings does it take to change a light bulb?

— None. That's what medical students are for.

A third year medical student was taking a long time with his first history and physical in the ER. Forty-five minutes into the interview, he got around to asking the patient if she was sexually active. She answered, "I might be if you'd hurry up and finish."

A third year medical student began doing a history and physical on an elderly man.

"Tell me," asked the student. "Do you suffer from arthritis?"

"Of course," snarled the old man. "What else can I do with it?"

How many pre-med students does it take to change a light bulb?

— Ten. One to change the bulb and nine to stand around and say, "I could have done that."

What's the difference between an undergraduate student, a graduate student, and a medical student?

— When the professor walks in and says, "Good morning class," the undergraduate says, "Good morning, Professor," the graduate student nods his head in acknowledgement, and the medical student writes it down.

(See also Case Presentations, History & Physical, Lectures, Physical Diagnosis, Roundsmanship, Scut)

~ MEDICARE ~

Show me a man who needs Medicare, and I'll show you a sick old man.
— *Anonymous* [(298)]

Medicare and Medicaid are the greatest measures yet devised to make the world safe for clerks.
— *Peter Drucker* [(247)]

A malpractice lawyer, an HMO administrator, and a Medicare auditor jump off the Empire State Building at the same time. Which one hits the ground first?
— Who cares?

How many Medicare auditors does it take to change a light bulb?
— Just one, but it really gets screwed.

Two elderly sisters go to see a new doctor. The doctor is a very thorough historian and asks the first one if she ever had gonorrhea. She says, "I don't know, let me ask my sister." The woman sticks her head in the next exam room and says, "Martha, have I ever had gonorrhea?" Her sister yells back, "I don't know, but if Medicare pays for it, get two!"

(See also Paperwork)

~ MEETINGS ~

(See Committees)

~ MEMORY ~

There are three signs of old age. One is loss of memory. The other two I forget.
— *Bob Hope* [(245)]

Calhoun's Law of Memory: You are more likely to remember something if you don't forget it.
— *Lawrence G. Calhoun, PhD, et al* [(80)]

"Don't worry about senility," my grandfather used to say. "When it hits you, you won't know it."
— *Bill Cosby* [135]

By the time you're 80 years old you've learned everything. You just have to remember it.
— *George Burns* [135]

My grandfather's a little forgetful, but he likes to give me advice. One day he took me aside and left me there.
— *Ron Richards* [184]

"Occasionally, I experience a complete loss of memory," Tracy said to her doctor. "What do you recommend?"

"I recommend you pay me in advance."

Two elderly gentlemen meet daily on a park bench to enjoy nature and to chat. One of them says to the other, "By the way, what's your name?" The other one answers, "How soon do you have to know?"

An 80-year-old's golf game was being hampered by poor eyesight. He could hit the ball well enough, but he couldn't see where it went. So his ophthalmologist teamed him up with another 80-year-old who had perfect eyesight and was willing to go along as a spotter.

The golfer hit the first ball and asked his companion if he saw where it landed.

"Yep," the man said.

"Where did it go?" the golfer asked.

The other man said, "I don't remember."

Two elderly couples were having a friendly conversation when one of the men said, "Fred, how was the memory clinic you went to last month?"

"Outstanding," said Fred. "They taught us all the latest techniques like visualization and association. It's made a huge difference for me."

"That's great," his friend said. "What was the name of the clinic?"

Fred went blank. He thought and thought, but couldn't remember the name. Then a smile spread across his face and he asked, "What do you call that red flower with the long stem and thorns?"

"You mean a rose?"

"Yeah, that's it." He turned to his wife, "Rose, what was the name of that clinic?"

Three old women were chatting at dinner. The first woman said, "You know, I'm getting really forgetful. This morning, I was standing at the top of the stairs, and I couldn't remember whether I had just come up or was about to go down."

The second woman said, "You think that's bad? The other day, I was sitting on the edge of my bed, and I couldn't remember whether I was going to sleep or had just woken up."

The third woman smiled smugly. "My memory is just as good as it's always been," she said, knocking on the table for good luck. She then looked up and said, "Who's there?"

(See also Alzheimer's Disease, Amnesia, Old Age)

~ MENOPAUSE ~

The symptoms of menopause in men—buying sports cars, dating teenagers, getting hair transplants—are not related to estrogen, but to stupidity.

— Mark DePaolis, MD [109]

A new study shows that menopausal women who are given testosterone not only experience an increase in energy, but they also start getting paid more.

— Dennis Miller [135]

Scientists have found a way to keep middle-aged female mice from going through menopause. Now they're working on a way to keep middle-aged male mice from buying expensive sports cars. *— Conan O'Brien* [135]

I'm trying very hard to understand this generation. They have adjusted the timetable for childbearing so that menopause and teaching a 16-year-old how to drive a car will occur in the same week. *— Erma Bombeck* [322]

~ MENSTRUATION ~

On menstruation:
Thank God it's a cycle and not something that increases exponentially.

— Garry Shandling [163]

There are three developmental stages in adolescent girls: pubarche, menarche, and anarchy.
— *Howard Bennett, MD* [48]

So what would happen if suddenly, magically, men could menstruate and women could not? Clearly, menstruation would become an enviable, boast-worthy masculine event . . . Congress would fund a National Institute of Dysmenorrhea . . . Sanitary supplies would be federally funded and free, though some men would still pay for the prestige of such commercial brands as Paul Newman Tampons, Muhammad Ali's Rope-a-Dope Pads, John Wayne Maxi Pads, and Joe Namath Jock Shields.
— *Gloria Steinem* [296]

(See also Gynecology, Pelvic Exam, PMS, Vagina)

~ Mental Status ~

Oriented X Three: A patient who is less confused than his physician.
— *Anonymous* [94]

The first thing to do at a psychiatric emergency is to check your own mental status.
— *Samuel Shem, MD* [282]

~ Microbiology ~

(See Bacteria)

~ Middle Age ~

Middle age is the time when a man is always thinking that in a week or two he will feel as good as ever.
— *Don Marquis* [125]

Middle age is that time of life when you can feel bad in the morning without having had fun the night before.
— *Anonymous* [2]

It's a sobering thought that when Mozart was my age, he had been dead for two years. — *Tom Lehrer* [196]

At 40 we are suddenly able to replace only the most important cells, like heart and small intestine cells, while things like knees and eyes have to fend for themselves. Fat cells do particularly well after 40, and our bodies will often try to use them as replacements for other parts, passing them off as a new chin or set of thigh muscles. — *Mark DePaolis, MD* [108]

You know you're getting older when the first thing you do after you're done eating is look for a place to lie down. — *Louis Anderson* [135]

After thirty, a body has a mind of its own. — *Bette Midler* [220]

One of the ironies of middle age is that as your waist gets thicker your hair gets thinner. — *Howard Bennett, MD* [48]

They say life begins at forty,
But with this I disagree—
That certainly isn't what happened
When forty caught up with me. — *Betty Grove Kitchen* [178]

Middle age is when you realize there's one more thing in the world that's biodegradable—you. — *Robert Orben* [184]

When you're over the hill, you pick up speed. — *Anonymous* [111]

Middle age is when you still believe you'll feel better in the morning. — *Anonymous* [135]

Middle age is when you're home on Saturday night and the telephone rings, and you hope it's a wrong number. — *Ring Lardner* [268]

My mind and body are going in the same direction, but not at the same speed. — *Margaret Randall* [197]

In a man's middle years there is scarcely a part of the body he would hesitate to turn over to the proper authorities.   — *E. B. White* [103]

Roses are red.
Violets are blue.
I'm middle-aged.
How about you?   — *Howard Bennett, MD* [48]

Middle age occurs when you are too young to take up golf and too old to rush the net.   — *Franklin P. Adams* [103]

After a serious accident, a woman lay in a coma. Her worried husband stood at her bedside for days. One afternoon the nurse said reassuringly, "Well, at least age is on her side."

"She's not so young," replied the husband. "She's forty-five."

At this point, the patient moved slightly and murmured, "Forty-four."

A middle-aged woman came back from a routine physical with a smile on her face.

"Why the grin?" asked her sour-faced husband.

"Because," she boasted, "Dr. Martin told me I have the bust of a woman half my age."

"Oh, yeah? And what about your 50-year-old ass?"

The woman answered, "Come to think of it, he didn't say a thing about you."

(See also Old Age)

~ MORBIDITY & MORTALITY CONFERENCE ~

If a chief resident runs an M&M conference for a year, his oral boards will assume the stress level of a goodnight kiss.   — *Leo A. Gordon, MD* [143]

"We couldn't find the films," means "We didn't care enough to steal the films."
                                                  — *Leo A. Gordon, MD* [143]

~ MOTHERHOOD ~

A suburban mother's role is to deliver children—obstetrically once and by car forever after.
— *Peter DeVries* [194]

It's not easy being a mother. If it was easy, fathers would do it.
— *Dorothy, "The Golden Girls"* [223]

I told my mother that I was thinking about seeing a therapist. She thought that was a good idea because she heard they make a lot of money.
— *Darlene Hunt* [67]

The phrase "working mother" is redundant.
— *Jane Sellman* [310]

I was on a corner the other day when a wild-looking, sort of gypsy-looking lady with a dark veil over her face grabbed me and said, "Karen Haber! You're never going to find happiness, and no one is ever going to marry you." I said, "Mom, leave me alone."
— *Karen Haber* [311]

The harried housewife ran to the phone when it rang and listened with relief to the kindly voice on the other end. "How are you darling?" it said. "What kind of day are you having?"

"Oh, mother," said the housewife breaking into tears. "I've had such an awful day. The baby won't eat and the washing machine broke down. I haven't had a chance to go shopping, and I just sprained my ankle. On top of that, the house is a mess and I'm supposed to have two couples over for dinner tonight."

The mother was at once all sympathy. "Oh, darling," she said, "sit down and relax. I'll be over in half an hour. I'll do the shopping, clean the house, and cook dinner for you. I'll feed the baby, and I'll call a repairman I know who'll be at your house to fix the washing machine right away. Now stop crying. I'll do everything. In fact, I'll even call George at the office and tell him he ought to come home and help out for once."

"George?" said the housewife. "Who's George?"

"Why, George, your husband! . . . Is this 555-1374?"

"No, it's 555-1375."

"Oh, I'm sorry. I guess I have the wrong number."

There was a short pause and the housewife said, "Does this mean you're not coming?"

(See also Babies, Biologic Clock, Children, Fatherhood, Parenting)

~ Multiple Personality Disorder ~

Dr. Niles Crane (on leaving the room): Well, this has been kind of fun, but I really must go. I'm conducting a seminar for multiple personality disorders, and it takes me forever to fill out the name tags.   — *"Frasier"* [131]

After six months of therapy, a psychiatrist was making excellent progress with a patient who had a multiple personality disorder. Since things were going so well, he decided to submit a bill for his services. Two weeks after he submitted the bill, the following letter arrived in the mail.

Dear Dr. Pierce:

As you will undoubtedly recall, Myra was the one responsible for initiating these sessions. She also did most of the talking during the past few months. Since we don't know where she is any more than you do, we have no intention of paying this bill.

Sincerely,
Beth, Laura, Pat & John

(See also Personality Disorder)

~ Mumps ~

If you get the mumps as a kid, you don't get 'em as an adult; but if you get 'em as an adult, you don't get kids.   — *Max Klinger, "M*A*S*H"* [200]

Between you and the mumps, Winchester, I prefer the mumps. At least I know they're going to go away.   — *Colonel Potter, "M*A*S*H"* [200]

~ Munchausen's Syndrome ~

From the Munchausen's Institute of America:
Impress your friends at parties. Fake an illness to get out of work. Baffle the experts at any medical center across the country. Call now for our free brochure: 1-800-THE BARON.

~ Murphy's Laws ~

- If anything can go wrong, it will.
- When anything goes wrong, it does so all at once.
- If two things can go wrong, the worst one will happen.
- If everything seems to be going well, you probably overlooked something.
- When left to themselves, things go from bad to worse.
- If it looks easy, it will be difficult. If it looks difficult, it will be damn near impossible.
- Nothing is ever as simple as it first seems.

(See also Aphorisms)

~ NEPHROLOGY ~

Homer Smith's Law: The function of the heart is to pump blood to the kidneys. [201]

Bock's Law: I pee, therefore I am. [135]

Lasix will squeeze urine out of bricks. — *Anonymous* [94]

A man spends the first 65 years of his life trying to make money; he spends the rest of it trying to make water. — *Robert Matz, MD* [246]

What do you get if you cross a librarian with a nephrologist?
— All the information you need, but it won't do you any good.

How many nephrologists does it take to change a light bulb?
— Two. One to screw in the bulb and the other to fill out an incident report for nicking the socket.

(See also Kidneys, Transplantation)

~ NEUROLOGY ~

Dead, adj. Deceased. Electroencephalographically challenged. — *Anonymous* [135]

Neurologic Definitions:
• Migraine: What a Russian farmer now says about his harvest.
• Pons: Popular facial cream.
• Sella: A good place to keep wine.
• Vertigo: How foreigners ask for directions.
• Porphyrins: Acquaintances who ask to borrow money.

Bloopers & Malapropisms:
- The left leg became numb at times and she walked it off.
- The patient is a healthy appearing 74-year-old white female, mentally alert but forgetful.
- The patient is a 68-year-old white male admitted to the VA hospital with aphasia and *downgrowing* toes. (downgoing)
- The patient's symptoms improved markedly once we initiated transcutaneous *nurse* stimulation. (nerve)
- Upon careful examination, it was noted that the infant had no *moral* reflex. (moro)
- Review of systems reveals a history of empty *cellar* syndrome. (sella)
- A 44-year-old man was admitted with a cerebral *conclusion*. (contusion)
- "Ever since my husband hurt his back, he's suffered with *Paris fevers* in his right foot." (paresthesias)
- She is numb from the toes down.
- The patient presented to the emergency room with weakness due to a transient *schematic* attack. (ischemic)
- The patient is a 85-year-old white male with *penile* dementia. (senile)
- My grandfather died of a cerebral *hemorrhoid*. (hemorrhage)
- The patient has low back pain and *ridiculitis*. (radiculitis)

Two doctors get lost in a hot air balloon when they see someone on the ground. They shout to the man, "Can you tell us where we are?"

The man looks up, thinks for a while, and says, "You're in a hot air balloon. You're about fifty feet off the ground, and you're located directly Southeast from where I'm standing."

One of the doctors in the balloon turns to the other and says, "He must be a neurologist."

"How can you tell?" his friend asks.

"Well, he thought about the problem carefully, his answer was amazingly accurate, but it didn't help us one bit."

Ross was sitting on the exam table in a well-known neurologist's office.

"Tell me," the neurologist said, "did you see anyone else before coming to me for this problem?"

"Yes," Ross said, "I saw my GP, Dr. Packer, last week."

"That quack!" the neurologist said. "And what advice did *he* give you?"

"He told me to come see you."

How many neurologists does it take to change a light bulb?
— Just one, but first he needs an EEG to make sure the old bulb is really dead.

(See also Brain, Headaches, Spine, Stroke)

~ Neurosurgery ~

Comment by a neurosurgeon who is also a night club singer:
I am much more comfortable in the operating room than on stage. If something goes wrong in surgery, the worst thing that can happen is you lose the patient.
— *Anonymous* [(211)]

A man who was having trouble with his sink called a plumber to his house. After the plumber checked the pipes, he leaned back and said, "I can fix the problem, but I want you to know that my fee is $200 per half hour."

"What!" said the startled man. "Why, I'm a neurosurgeon, and I only get $200 for a full hour."

"Hey, don't feel bad," the plumber said sympathetically. "When I was a neurosurgeon, I only made $200 an hour myself."

What's the difference between God and a neurosurgeon?
— God doesn't think he's a neurosurgeon.

How many neurosurgeons does it take to change a light bulb?
— Who knows, it's never been done.

~ Neurotics ~

I'm not co-dependent myself, but aren't they great to have around?
— *Betsy Salkind* [(135)]

Neurotic means he is not as sensible as I am, and psychotic means he's even worse than my brother-in-law. — *Karl Menninger, MD* [(103)]

I have an intense desire to return to the womb. Anybody's. — *Woody Allen* [(268)]

A neurotic is a person who, when you ask him how he is, tells you.
— *Anonymous* [(71)]

(See also Anxiety, Phobias, Stress)

~ Night Call ~

According to a recent study published in the *Annals of Nightcall*, only 5% of the calls that come in at night are truly urgent. The other 95% can be broken down into the following categories:
• Questions that could have waited till morning.
• Questions that could have waited till the patient's regular doc got back from vacation.
• Questions that could have waited till the end of time. — *Howard Bennett, MD* [44]

Peter, Peter, overeater
The nurses think he needs a sleeper;
At 2AM they call Doc Jake.
Now Pete's asleep and Jake's awake. — *Kim Shaftner, MD* [277]

When I chose to become a physician
I was following family tradition.
  But had I a peep
  Of how little I'd sleep,
I might have become a musician. — *Howard Bennett, MD* [41]

Ratner's Law: Beepers work better if you turn them on. [135]

What are answering service operators top five pet peeves?
• Patients with multiple personalities who call in six times for the same complaint.
• Digital headsets that keep picking up *Jerry Springer*.
• Choking patients who garble their phone number.
• Working the night shift, but not getting to wake anybody up.
• Prank calls from ex-coworkers who now have really good jobs that *don't* involve working with doctors.

The phone rang at Dr. Jackson's house as he sat down to dinner. He answered the call, listened for a moment, and then slammed down the receiver. "Quick, get my bag and car keys. There's a man on the phone who says he can't live without me."
  Jackson's daughter rolled her eyes. "Daddy, I believe that call was for me."

(See also Beepers, Caffeine, House Calls, Medical Practice)

~ Nose Jobs ~

You can hardly pick up a paper nowadays without the story of some prominent person having the contour of his or her nose reassembled. In the old days you used to be born with an appendix and a nose, and you went through life practically ignorant of the shape of either.
— *Will Rogers* [20]

Some girls insist on fancy cars,
Like Cadillacs and Jaguars,
Or they want men with big chateaus—
All I want's a little nose.
— *Lilly E. Carlton* [82]

The technical term for the nose job is *rhinoplasty*. Rhino? I mean, do we really need to insult the person at this particular moment in their life? They know they have a big nose, that's why they're coming in.
— *Jerry Seinfeld* [275]

~ Nurses ~

After two days in the hospital, I took a turn for the nurse.
— *W. C. Fields* [29]

Half a nurse is better than none.
— *Howard Bennett, MD* [48]

Having to work the night shift is like sex. You're always wondering when it will happen and how long it will last.
— *Anonymous* [135]

There once was a floor nurse named Doodle
Who rarely relied on her noodle.
    When temperatures rose
    She powdered her nose
And sat on her kit and caboodle.
— *Howard Bennett, MD* [41]

Once, while convalescing in the hospital, Dorothy Parker wanted to dictate some letters to her secretary. Before they set to work, she pressed the nurse's button and said, "This should assure us of at least 45 minutes of undisturbed privacy." [116]

A nurse called a resident at 3 AM. "Come quick," she said. "Your patient, Mrs. Parks, just swallowed a thermometer."

The resident hung up the phone and put on his jacket, but before he could get out the door the nurse called back.

"Never mind," she said. "I found another one."

How many doctors does it take to change a light bulb?
— Only one, but he has to have a nurse to tell him which end to screw in.

How many nurses does it take to change a lightbulb?
— Four. One to change the bulb, one to check the policy and procedure manual, one for documentation, and one for quality assurance.

A nurse had dinner with a friend after work. She paid the bill with a credit card, but when she reached into her pocket for a pen, she pulled out a rectal thermometer.

"Damn," she said. "Some asshole's got my pen."

(See also Hospitals)

~ NURSING HOMES ~

Nursing home doctors are always wrong. *— Paddy Chayefsky* [86]

Law #5 of the House of God—Placement Comes First. *— Samuel Shem, MD* [281]

Be nice to your children. After all, they are going to choose your nursing home.
— Steven Wright [135]

Fever spike: Something that happens the night before a patient is scheduled for nursing home placement. *— Rip Pfeiffer, MD* [248]

We are a long-term care facility, Mrs. Williams, which means that over the long term you will get some care. *— Peter Steiner* [61]

Dr. Parks drove to a nursing home to make rounds on his 99-year-old patient, Mr. Ward. After finishing the examination, the doctor said, "I fully expect to see you celebrate your one hundredth birthday."

"No reason why you shouldn't," Mr. Ward said. "You look pretty healthy to me."

An elderly male resident in a nursing home bet one of his female companions that she couldn't guess how old he was. She replied, "I can if you take off all your clothes."

So the man disrobed and she instructed him to turn around slowly. After a few minutes, she stroked her chin and said, "You're ninety-five."

"That's amazing!" he exclaimed. "How could you tell?"

"You told me at breakfast."

How many nursing home doctors does it take to change a light bulb?
— Just one, but he won't get around to it till the end of the month.

(See also Hearing, Memory, Old Age)

~ NUTRITION ~

(See Food)

O

~ Obesity ~

A lot of people have the "right stuff" but too many of those who have it, have it in the wrong places. — *Anonymous* [219]

The Krebs Cycle is a series of complicated biochemical reactions that show how everything we eat turns to fat. — *Howard Bennett, MD* [48]

At 40 we are suddenly able to replace only the most important cells, like heart and small intestine cells, while things like knees and eyes have to fend for themselves. Fat cells do particularly well after 40, and our bodies will often try to use them as replacements for other parts, passing them off as a new chin or set of thigh muscles. — *Mark DePaolis, MD* [108]

Being overweight is less often caused by an underactive metabolism than an overactive fork. — *John G. Hipps, MD* [158]

Fatty tissue looks like jelly.
Most is found around the belly.
All the rest (it seems unfair)
Decorates the derriere. — *Michael M. Stewart, MD* [297]

As part of its truth-in-labeling campaign, the Food and Drug Administration just announced that cellulite would be officially renamed, cellulard.
— *Ludwig Lettau, MD* [246]

A new study shows that three quarters of all Americans are overweight. In fact, it's so bad that three quarters of all Americans are nine-tenths of all Americans.
— *Conan O'Brien* [135]

Obesity is the mother of distension. — *Howard Bennett, MD* [48]

The stigma of being fat is nothing compared to that of being a smoker. If a fat person eats a double burrito, that burrito is history. There is no talk about second-hand cholesterol from the refried beans causing heart disease among passers-by. — *Michael Robertson* [259]

Ralph Kramden (on a new scheme): I'm tellin' you Alice, this is probably the biggest thing I've ever gotten into.
Alice Kramden: Ralph, the biggest thing you've ever gotten into is your pants.
— *"The Honeymooners"* [161]

I see no objection to stoutness, in moderation. — *Sir William S. Gilbert* [298]

Hot Lips Houlihan: Frank, you have a fat, fat princess.
Frank Burns: That just means there's more of you to love.
Hot Lips: So you agree I'm fat?
Frank: No Margaret, not fat-fat. You're sort of halfway between fat and thin, leaning a little bit to the not fat but rather the thin side of fat.
— *"M*A*S*H"* [200]

An obese woman got on a crowded bus. She stood in the aisle, looked around, and said, "Isn't anyone going to give me a seat?"
A thin man stood up and said, "I'll be glad to make a contribution."

A doctor finished examining his patient and began to talk with him. "Mr. Strauss, I find very little wrong with you. You're in surprisingly good health given your overweight condition. My advice is that you give up those intimate little dinners for two until you find another person to eat with."

(See also Dieting, Food, Liposcution)

~ Obsessive-Compulsive Behavior ~

I can't help it. I like things clean. Blame it on my mother. I was toilet trained when I was five months old. — *Felix Unger, "The Odd Couple"* [233]

Dr. Frasier Crane (to a caller): And while I agree that washing his hands twenty to thirty times a day would be considered obsessive-compulsive behavior, bear in mind that your husband *is* a coroner.   — *"Frasier"* (131)

There was a young lady of Crete,
Who was so exceedingly neat,
  When she got out of bed
  She stood on her head,
To make sure of not soiling her feet.   — *Anonymous* (308)

(See also Personality Disorders)

~ OBSTETRICS ~

My wife and I had all the complications you'd expect at a doctor's delivery—the epidural didn't work, they had to use forceps, and my mother-in-law stayed for three weeks.   — *Ryan James, MD* (246)

Cama's Law: Pitocin is good, but forceps are better. (135)

Little Miss Muffet
Decided to rough it
By shooing the drugs away.
Then came a contraction,
That caused a retraction,
And "Bradley" was quickly passé.   — *Howard Bennett, MD* (47)

An epidural is a needle you put in a woman's back that makes her numb from the waist down . . . for years.   — *Chip Franklin* (135)

A sign hanging in the OB ward of a hospital:
Research shows that the first five minutes of life can be the most risky.
Underneath someone had scrawled: The last five minutes aren't so great either. (135)

Bloopers & Malapropisms:

- The patient went into premature labor because of an incompetent *service*. (cervix)
- At the time of onset of pregnancy the mother was undergoing bronchoscopy.
- The patient was rushed to the delivery room because of *fecal* distress. (fetal)
- A healthy 8 pound girl was born after an uncomplicated *tern* pregnancy. (term)
- The patient has had two abortions and one *atopic* pregnancy. (ectopic)
- The patient says she is going through her *mental pause*. (menopause)
- Mrs. Johnston is scheduled for an ultrasound for *illegal hydramnios*. (oligo-hydramnios)
- A woman who was eight months pregnant called to say she was having *erotic* contractions. (erratic)
- After I had my third child, I decided to get a tubal *litigation*. (ligation)

(See also Birth Control, Childbirth, Condoms, C-Sections, Gynecology, Infertility, Pregnancy, Vagina)

~ OLD AGE ~

There are only three things you need to know about getting old. One is that you forget things, and the other two I don't remember.   — *William Kannel, MD* [171]

A man is as old as his arteries.   — *Thomas Sydenham* [298]

I've got everything I always had, only now it's six inches lower.
    — *Gypsy Rose Lee* [195]

My parents moved to Florida this year. They didn't want to move, but they're in their sixties and that's the law.   — *Jerry Seinfeld* [275]

There are three ages of man: youth, middle age, and "Gee, you look good."
    — *Red Skelton* [96]

I'm in the prime of my senility.   — *Benjamin Franklin* [125]

Senescence begins and middle age ends
The day your descendants outnumber your friends.   — *Ogden Nash* [217]

You know you're getting older when you wake up with that morning-after feeling, and you didn't do anything the night before.   — *Lois L. Kaufman* [184]

At my age, I need all the preservatives I can get.   — *George Burns* [268]

A man is only as old as the woman he feels.   — *Groucho Marx* [247]

You know you're getting old when "getting lucky" means you've found your car in the parking lot.   — *Bruce Lansky* [184]

I am just turning forty and taking my time about it.
— *Harold Lloyd, when asked his age at 77* [103]

My wife never lies about her age. She just tells people she's as old as I am. Then she lies about my age.   — *Anonymous* [135]

Anyone can get old. All you have to do is live long enough.   — *Grouch Marx* [268]

First you forget names, then you forget faces; then you forget to pull your zipper up, then you forget to pull your zipper down.   — *Leo Rosenberg* [247]

Very, very, very few
People die at ninety-two.
I suppose that I shall be
Safer still at ninety-three.   — *Willard R. Espy* [217]

There is something to be said for growing old. Not much, but something.
— *Laura Black* [54]

Age is a question of mind over matter. If you don't mind, it doesn't matter.
— *Satchel Paige* [321]

The secret of staying young is to live honestly, eat slowly, and lie about your age. — *Lucille Ball* [321]

I used to dread getting older because I thought I would not be able to do all the things I wanted to do, but now that I am older, I find that I don't want to do them. — *Nancy Astor* [68]

To me, old age is always fifteen years older than I am. — *Bernard Baruch* [103]

If you live to the age of a hundred, you've got it made because very few people die past the age of a hundred. — *George Burns* [268]

My diseases are an asthma and a dropsy and, what is less curable, seventy-five. — *Samuel Johnson* [219]

"I'm eighty years old, but I can only have sex once a month," George Burns said to his doctor.

"That's normal," his doc said.

"Maybe so," Burns complained, "but Groucho Marx is eighty-five and he says he has sex twice a week."

"Okay," replied the doctor, "you say the same thing."

An old man went to see his doctor for a checkup. At the end of the visit the doctor said, "I think you should cut your sex life in half."

"Which half," the man said, "talking about it or thinking about it?"

An elderly man decided to get married again. The couple wanted to have a baby, but they had no luck so the man went to get his sperm count checked.

After doing a history and physical examination, the doctor handed the man a jar. "Take this home and bring a sample back in the morning."

The old man returned with an empty jar. "I tried," he said wearily. "I tried with my left hand. Nothing. I tried with my right hand. Nothing. I tried with both hands. Nothing. I asked my wife. She tried with both hands. Nothing. We even asked the lady across the street to try, but she couldn't do it either."

"You asked your neighbor?" the doctor asked incredulously.

"Yes," the old man said. "None of us could get the lid off that jar."

A 80-year-old man went to see his doctor for a routine checkup.

"Doc," the octogenarian said, "my wife, who is eighteen, is about to have a baby.

"Really?" the doctor said.

"Really," the man answered.

"Let me tell you a story," the doctor said. "A man went hunting, but instead of taking his gun, he picked up an umbrella by mistake. When a bear suddenly charged at him, he pointed his umbrella at the bear, shot, and killed it on the spot."

"That's impossible," the old man said. "Somebody else must have shot that bear."

"Exactly my point."

(See also Alzheimer's Disease, Geriatrics, Hearing Loss, Longevity, Memory, Middle Age, Nursing Homes)

~ ONCOLOGY ~

(See Cancer)

~ OPHTHALMOLOGY ~

Sign on an ophthalmologist's door:
If you don't see what you want, you've come to the right place. [135]

Ophthalmology Definitions:
• Blind spot: A dog that can't see.
• Dilate: Live a long life.
• Fundus: A grant application plea.
• Unreactive pupil: Resident after a rough night on call.
— *Robert C. Scott, MD & W. Michael Myles, MD* [274]

Bloopers & Malapropisms:
• The fundiscopic exam did not reveal *papal edema*. (papilledema)
• The patient developed a swollen right eye, which was felt to be secondary to an insect bite by an ophthalmologist.

• Past medical history reveals surgery for a *regular blastoma*. (retinoblastoma)
• The patient has a history of *immaculate* degeneration. (macular)
• Examination revealed a *high femur* of the right eye. (hyphema)

Did you hear about the nearsighted old woman? In order to hide her failing eyesight from her son, she decided to trick him. One afternoon, she stuck a daisy in a tree. The next day, while walking in a meadow with her son, she pointed to the tree, some fifty yards away, and said, "Isn't that a daisy sticking out of that tree?" And as she ran to retrieve it, she tripped over a cow.

An 80-year-old's golf game was being hampered by poor eyesight. He could hit the ball well enough, but he couldn't see where it went. So his ophthalmologist teamed him up with another 80-year-old who had perfect eyesight and was willing to go along as a spotter.

The golfer hit the first ball and asked his companion if he saw where it landed.

"Yep," the man said.

"Where did it go?" the golfer asked.

The other man said, "I don't remember."

Dr. Krauss performed a delicate eye operation and restored the vision of a famous painter. As a gesture of thanks, the artist presented Dr. Krauss with a portrait of the ophthalmologist inside a giant eyeball.

Dr. Krauss brought the painting home and showed it to his wife. "What do you think?" he asked.

After looking at it for a long time his wife said, "I'm glad I didn't marry a proctologist."

"Miss Ryan," said the anatomy teacher, "would you please tell the class what part of the body enlarges to five times its normal size during periods of agitation or emotional excitement?"

Blushing, the woman said, "Professor, I would rather not answer that question."

Raising a brow, the professor asked, "Oh? And why not?"

"Well, sir, it's kind of personal."

"Not at all," he blustered. "The correct answer is the pupil of the eye, and your response tells me two things. First, you didn't read last night's assignment. And second, marriage is going to leave you a tremendously disappointed young woman."

(See also Glasses)

~ ORTHOPEDICS ~

Heart, n. A muscular pump whose sole purpose is to get antibiotics into the bones.
— *Anonymous* [94]

Traction speaks louder than words.
— *Howard Bennett, MD* [48]

On visiting a friend who just had a hip replaced:
What's a nice joint like that doing in a guy like you?
— *Herb Caen* [78]

Orthopod's Spot: By placing the stethoscope on the xiphoid process you can simultaneously auscultate the heart, lungs, and bowels.
— *Anonymous* [248]

Orthopedic Definitions:
• Carpal: Someone you drive to work with.
• Castrate: The going price for setting a fracture.
• Currette: A partial recovery.
• Fibula: A little white lie.
• Dislocation: Here.

Bloopers & Malapropisms:
• On the second day the knee was better, and on the third day it had completely disappeared.
• A 4-year-old girl fell and broke her wrist. When her mom got the name of an orthopedist who would cast the fracture, the girl said, "Why do I have to see an orthopenis?"
• A week after surgery, she spiked a *femur*. (fever)

How can you tell the difference between an internist and an orthopedist when they're rushing to get on an elevator?
— The internist holds the door open with his hands; the orthopod uses his head.

How can you hide a $100 bill from an orthopod?
— Put it in a book.

What are the two best years in an orthopedist's life?
— Second grade.

What's the difference between a gorilla and an orthopedist?
— One is hairy and strong and communicates with a series of grunts, and the other one lives in a zoo.

How many orthopedists does it take to change a light bulb?
— Two. One to force it in with a hammer and the other to ask the circulating nurse for a new bulb.

A lawyer's wife broke her hip on a skiing trip. The lawyer got the best orthopedist in town to do the procedure. The operation consisted of lining up the fractured bone and putting in two screws to secure it. The operation was a success, and the doctor sent the lawyer a bill for $5000. The lawyer was shocked at the charges and sent the doctor a letter demanding an explanation for the costs. The orthopedist sent back the following note:

2 screws: $1.
Knowing how to put them in: $4999.

(See also Arthritis, Backache, Club Foot, Exercise, Fractures, Jogging, Knees, Spine, Sports Medicine, X-Rays)

~ OSTEOPATHS ~

An osteopath is someone who argues that all human ills are caused by the pressure of hard bone upon soft tissue. The proof of this theory can be found in the heads of those who believe it.   — *H. L. Mencken* [71]

~ OTOLARYNGOLOGY ~

(See Ear, Nose & Throat)

P

~ PAIN ~

When doctors describe pain as experiencing "discomfort," it's like saying Hiroshima experienced "urban renewal."   — *Dave Barry* [25]

There once was a "healer" from Deal,
Who said, "Although pain isn't real,
   If I sit on a pin
   And it punctures my skin,
I dislike what I fancy I feel."

— *Anonymous* [103]

~ PANCREAS ~

I'm tired of all this nonsense about beauty being only skin deep. That's deep enough. What do you want an adorable pancreas?   — *Jean Kerr* [135]

God put the pancreas in the back because he didn't want surgeons messin' with it.   — *Rip Pfeiffer, MD* [248]

~ PAPERWORK ~

In the past, we took off Wednesday afternoons for 18 holes of golf. Now we take off Wednesday afternoons for 18 hours of paperwork.

— *Stu Silverstein, MD* [246]

On doing paperwork:
I usually approach this task like a child eating spinach: there are new piles every few minutes, but nothing disappears.   — *Howard Bennett, MD* [43]

Life is short and vacations are shorter, but paperwork is eternal.

— Howard Bennett, MD [(40)]

~ PARANOID ~

(See Personality Disorders)

~ PARENTING ~

The way I look at it, if my kids are still alive at the end of the day, I've done my job.

— Rosanne Barr [(135)]

For me, parenting is like dieting. Every day, I wake up filled with resolve and good intentions, perfection in view, and every day I somehow stray from the path. The difference is, with dieting I usually make it to lunch.

— Marion Winik [(319)]

There are three stages in a parent's life—nutrition, dentition, and tuition.

— Marcelene Cox [(195)]

We're pretty strict about sleep habits in my house. The only thing that's allowed to wake me up at 5AM is my bladder.

— Howard Bennett, MD [(48)]

Kids aren't easy, but there has to be some penalty for sex.

— Bill Maher [(135)]

Whenever my first child dropped his pacifier, I boiled it to make sure it was clean. Now that I have three kids, if anyone drops a pacifier I let the dog pick it up.

— Molly Ryan, MD [(246)]

It's illegal in forty-seven states to leave a child in a rest room during a family vacation and pretend it was a mistake.

— Erma Bombeck [(135)]

In America there are two classes of travel—first class, and with children.

— Robert Benchley [(96)]

For years, my husband and I advocated separate vacations. But the kids kept finding us. — *Erma Bombeck* [195]

I never understood why late afternoon is called "Arsenic Hour." Are you supposed to take it yourself or give it to your kids? — *Mandy Katz* [246]

Bruce Springsteen has kids and he doesn't give those 4 hour concerts anymore. After an hour and a half, he says, "Are you ready to rock and roll?" And the audience answers, "No, Bruce, we've got sitters." And he says, "Oh, shit, me too. Goodnight." — *Paul Clay* [67]

As parents, my wife and I have one thing in common. We're both afraid of children. — *Bill Cosby* [245]

I used to worry about losing my husband to another woman. Now, I'm more afraid of losing my nanny to another woman. — *Sybil Adelman* [3]

Psychologists say that children act out at home because they love their parents and feel safe letting out their negative energy. Hell, if my kids love me any more, I'll need a frontal lobotomy. — *Howard Bennett, MD* [48]

When you go from two to three children, it's important that you switch from a man-to-man to a zone defense. — *Mandy Katz* [246]

Parenting requires patience, endurance, forgiveness, understanding. And if the children aren't willing to do that, it's going to be tough. — *Gene Perret* [245]

The thing to remember about fathers is, they're men. — *Phyllis McGinley* [197]

It goes without saying that you should never have more children than you have car windows. — *Erma Bombeck* [135]

The law of heredity is that all undesirable traits come from the other parent. — *Anonymous* [103]

Any child will run any errand for you, if you ask at bedtime. — *Red Skelton* [218]

Human beings are the only creatures that allow their children to come back home.
                                                      — *Bill Cosby* [163]

The best way to give advice to your children is to find out what they want and then advise them to do it.   — *Harry S. Truman* [217]

Children are unpredictable. You never know that inconsistency they're going to catch you in next.   — *Franklin P. Jones* [247]

Before I got married I had six theories about bringing up children. Now I have six children and no theories.   — *John Wilmot* [247]

Children are a great comfort in old age—and they help you reach if faster too.
                                                   — *Lionel Kauffman* [247]

An 8-year-old girl was talking with her grandmother when the subject of discipline came up. "When I was a young girl," the old woman said, "my father used to spank me."
    "Really?" the girl said. "My dad doesn't believe in spanking."
    "What does he do instead?" the grandmother asked.
    "Oh, he just makes a speech about things."
    "And what does he say?" the grandmother asked.
    "Search me," the girl answered. "I never listen."

The parents of a 2-year-old were worried because their child had never uttered a word. They took her to a handful of specialists, but no one found anything wrong with the child.
    When the child was three, she still hadn't spoken a word. Then, a week before her fourth birthday, her father put a plate of chicken, mashed potatoes, and spinach in front of her.
    The child pushed the plate away and said, "I hate spinach."
    The father was astonished and called his wife into the kitchen. "Megan," he said, "tell you mother what you just told me."
    "I hate spinach," the child repeated.
    The parents went crazy, laughing and dancing around the child with delight.
    When they finally calmed down, the mother said, "We're so happy you can talk Megan, but why has it taken so long for you to say anything to us?"
    The child said, "Up till now, everything's been okay."

On the first day of school, a first grader handed his teacher a note from his mother. It said, "The opinions expressed by this child are not necessarily those of his parents."

(See also Babies, Biologic Clock, Children, Fatherhood, Heredity, Motherhood)

~ Pathology ~

An internist is someone who knows everything and does nothing. A surgeon is someone who knows nothing and does everything. A pathologist is someone who knows everything and does everything but too late. — *Anonymous* [94]

A medical examiner is a coroner with a bigger office. — *Ryan James, MD* [246]

Bloopers & Malapropisms:
• The patient had never been fatally ill before.
• The patient went to bed feeling perfectly normal, but woke up dead.
• I just finished the autopsy on your father, and I can tell you that he didn't die of anything serious.
• The patient expired on the floor uneventfully.
• The emergency room doctor suspected suicide, but the patient later denied this.

Four doctors went duck hunting—an internist, a radiologist, a surgeon, and a pathologist. As they crouched in the grass, they agreed to let the internist shoot first. The first flock of birds approached and the internist raised his shotgun toward the sky. With a puzzled look on his face, he lowered his gun, only to raise it again as the ducks flew off. When his colleagues inquired why he didn't shoot, the internist replied, "When they were coming toward me, they looked like ducks. Then I looked again and thought they were geese. By the time I was sure they were ducks, they were gone." Next up was the radiologist. As the ducks flew towards the hunters, the barrel was raised and once again it was lowered. As the birds flew away the radiologist shook his head in frustration. "They looked like ducks in the lateral view, but I couldn't be sure until I saw the PA view. By then, they were gone." Next up was the surgeon. As the birds approached, he began firing wildly in all directions. Ducks fell from the sky like rain. When the smoke cleared, the surgeon gathered up all of the fallen fowl and handed them to the pathologist. "Here," he said triumphantly, "let me know what these are?"

What's the definition of a pathologist?
— Someone who washes his hands *before* he goes to the bathroom.

(See also Autopsy, Coroner)

~ Patients & Patient Care ~

When I first started out in practice, I lied awake at night worrying about my patients. Now I lie awake worrying about their lawyers.   — *Howard Fischer, MD* [246]

Chronic, adj. Describing an entity that will not go away, despite the doctor's best efforts; sometimes a disease, often a patient.
— *George Thomas, MD & Lee Schreiner, MD* [303]

The Law of Discharge: Any labs done on the day of discharge will be abnormal.
— *Anonymous* [135]

If you tell a patient to lie down, he will almost always lie on his back; if you tell him to lie on his back, he will almost always lie on his stomach.
— *Anonymous* [94]

How to be a professional patient:
• Never call the doctor during the day if a night call will do.
• Make the doctor extract the history. Remember, you're paying him.
• Take your time. The doctor is probably in more of a hurry than you are.
— *Ian Rose, MD* [265]

On the proper frame of mind before undergoing surgery:
Console yourself with the reflection that you are giving the doctor pleasure, and that he is getting paid for it.   — *Mark Twain* [19]

No-show patients never have the last appointment of the day.
— *Patrick J. Taylor, MD* [301]

What to say to patients when things aren't going as planned:
Medicine is an art, not a science.   — *Anne Eva Ricks, MD* [256]

Rules patients should follow to keep their doctors happy:
• Try to suffer from the disease for which you are being treated.
• Don't ask your doctor if he knows what he is doing.
• Don't ask for a second opinion.
• Don't suffer from ailments that you cannot afford.
• Don't die in your doctor's presence. — *Anonymous* [135]

Old Mother Hubbard,
Went to be cultured,
Cause it hurt when she swallowed a scone.
But when she got there,
The wait was a bear,
So Old Mother Hubbard went home. — *Howard Bennett, MD* [45]

It's hard work becoming a patient. First of all, you have to get sick, which usually happens at night. Then, if you're lucky enough to survive till morning, you still have to make an appointment to see the doctor. — *Rick Stevens, MD* [246]

Patients need doctors for two reasons: First, to get sound medical advice on how to treat their condition. And second, to have someone to blame in case things don't get better. — *Mark DePaolis, MD* [109]

Balluff's Constant of Memory:
• The number of medications a patient takes are inversely proportional to the patient's ability to remember what those medications are.
• Corollary No. 1: The patient will always describe the medication he cannot remember as "a little white pill."
• Corollary No. 2: If a patient says, "My wife knows what medicines I take," the wife will not have a clue. [101]

What are the most common reasons patients give for being late to an appointment:
• By mistake, they went to the office of the other Herbert T. Slotnick in your building.
• They got held up waiting in line to buy the new bestseller, "Patients Who Complain Too Much and the Doctors Who Avoid Them."
• Two of their six personalities refused to get dressed that morning.
• They lost track of time watching *As the World Turns*.

What do you call nonpaying patients?
— Relatives.

A middle-aged woman came back from her physical with a smile on her face.

"Why the grin?" asked her sour faced husband.

"Because," she boasted, "Dr. Martin told me I have the bust of a woman half my age."

"Oh, yeah? And what about your 50-year-old ass?"

The woman answered, "Come to think of it, he didn't say a thing about you."

(See also Advice, Compliance, Doctor-Patient Communication, Hospitals, House Calls, Hypochondriacs, Procedures)

~ PEARLS ~

Today's pearl is tomorrow's fecalith.
— Daniel J. Waters, DO [312]

A pearl is a nugget of wisdom bestowed by an attending to a grateful medical student—right before he asks him to do some scut. *— Howard Bennett, MD* [40]

(See also Roundsmanship, Scut)

~ PEDIATRICS ~

Never trust a naked baby.
— Anonymous [94]

The best way to stop a child's cough is to make an appointment to see the doctor.
— Larry Bauer, MD [246]

Pediatricians eat because children don't.
— Meyer A. Perlstein, MD [298]

The only way to keep a child from ingesting a drug is to prescribe it for him.
— David Guttman, MD [151]

In pediatrics, the vaccine schedule always gets a little behind.
— Ludwig Lettau, MD [246]

There are only two things a child will share willingly—communicable diseases
and his mother's age. — *Benjamin Spock, MD* [293]

Apnea, n. Form of greeting to one whose arrival has been unduly delayed; as
"We was wondering what apnea." — *H.S. Grannatt* [144]

The difference between a pediatrician and an internist is how you feel when
your patient pees on you. — *Andy Biles* [135]

Bloopers & Malapropisms:
• This newborn infant has an incomplete *moral* reflex. (moro)
• Chief complaint: 3-year-old with a *postnavel* drip. (postnasal)
• "My son just drank some mouthwash. Should we give him *ipecat*?" (ipecac)
• I asked a 4-year-old to take off his underpants so I could examine his penis.
  He said, "I don't have any peanuts."
• The infant was handed to the pediatrician, who cried spontaneously.
• After an extensive evaluation, it was determined that the diagnosis was
  Munchkin's by Proxy. (Munchausen's)
• The patient is an 8-year-old boy who presents with a two week history of large
  lymph *nose*. (nodes)
• The patient has a history of constipation and rectal *fishers*. (fissures)

How many neonatologists does it take to change a light bulb?
— Just one, but the bulb has to be less than 15 watts.

(See also Babies, Bedwetting, Behavior Management, Breast Feeding,
Children, Circumcision, Conjunctivitis, Diapers, Fever, Foreign Body, Mumps,
Parenting, Spinal Tap, Teeth, Thumb Sucking, Toilet Training, Umbilical Cord)

~ PELVIC EXAMS ~

On comparing pelvic and rectal exams:
Women have been having things like this done every year with very little whining, which is just another reason to be glad they are the ones giving birth. Given
the choice, many men would simply say, "I hate this part," and the human
species would never reproduce. — *Mark DePaolis, MD* [108]

Recognizing the importance of ethical issues in medicine, Dr. Marcus always insisted on the presence of a third party whenever he examined a female patient.

Near the end of a busy afternoon, the doctor wearily motioned a couple into the examination room. The woman complained of pains in her lower abdomen and submitted to a pelvic exam reluctantly. The man looked on with interest.

When he finished, the doctor prescribed some medication and the woman jumped up from the table, dressed hurriedly, and ran from the room.

"Your wife certainly is edgy," the doctor said. "She'll be all right in a few days."

"My wife?" said the man. "I've never seen her before, doc. I was wondering why you called me in here."

(See also Gynecology)

~ Penis ~

My 3-year-old is so enamored of his penis these days that he can't do anything that requires two hands.
— *Molly Ryan, MD* [246]

Science magazine came out with a report on the difference between men's and women's brains. Apparently women are controlled by a part of the brain called the cingulate gyrus and men are controlled by a part of the brain known as the penis.
— *Jay Leno* [135]

Annie Hall (after a visit to her psychiatrist): Then she mentioned penis envy. Do you know about that?
Alvy Singer: Me? I'm one of the few males who suffer from that.
— *Woody Allen & Marshall Brickman, "Annie Hall"* [9]

After three years in analysis, a patient had her last therapy session with Sigmund Freud. On leaving the office, the patient turned to the celebrated doctor with a puzzled look on her face. Noting her expression, Freud said, "Do you have a question my dear?"

"Why yes, Herr Freud, I do. After all these years in therapy, I'm still not sure what a phallus is."

At this point, Freud escorted the woman back into his office, pulled down his trousers and pointed between his legs. "This, my dear, is a phallus."

"Oh, I see," said the patient. "It's like a penis . . . only smaller."

(See also Circumcision, Masturbation, Urology, Venereal Disease)

~ PERSONALITY DISORDERS ~

It's unethical to diagnose patients as borderline just because they're having more fun than you are. *— Joel Herscovitch, PhD* [156]

The true paranoid is the one in possession of all the facts. *— Anonymous* [135]

Just because you're paranoid doesn't mean you're not being followed. *— Anonymous* [103]

Did you hear about the narcissistic opera singer?
— Her favorite aria was, "Mi, Mi, Mi, Mi."

(See also Multiple Personality Disorder, Neurotics, Obsessive-Compulsive Behavior)

~ PHARMACISTS ~

Mrs. Altman sent an invitation to her internist asking if he'd like to attend a dinner party she was having. The internist sent back his reply in a timely manner, but the note was completely illegible. "I don't know if he accepted or refused," she told a friend. "I can't read the note."

"Take it to a pharmacy," her friend advised. "No matter how badly my doctor writes his prescriptions, the druggist always seems to be able to read it."

Mrs. Altman followed her friend's advice. The druggist looked at the note, disappeared into the back room and returned a few minutes later with a small bottle.

"Here you are," he said. "That will be thirty-five dollars."

An attractive young woman got caught in a sudden rainstorm. By the time she got under cover, she was drenched and needed a cigarette. A friend standing nearby reached into her pocket and pulled out a small rubber thing, unrolled it, and took out a perfectly dry cigarette. It was in a condom.

The woman said, "That's a great idea. I'll have to try it."

So the next day the woman went to a drugstore and said, "A package of condoms, please."

"What kind?" asked the pharmacist.

"I'm not sure," the woman said, "I guess it should be big enough for a Camel."

A man rushed into a drug store and said to the pharmacist, "Do you have anything that will stop hiccups?"

The pharmacist leaned over the counter and slapped the man in the face.

"Why the heck did you do that?" the man said.

"It stopped your hiccups didn't it?"

"I don't have the hiccups, you dumbbell. My wife does, and she's in the car."

(See also Drug Stores)

~ PHOBIAS ~

Tell us your phobias and we'll tell you what you are afraid of.

— *Robert Benchley* [116]

~ PHYSICAL DIAGNOSIS ~

The most important sign is the one no one else has found.   — *Ian Rose, MD* [264]

On when to get a routine check-up:
Extensive medical research has shown that there is only one reliable sign that it is time for men to see a doctor—when their wives make them go.

— *Mark DePaolis, MD* [108]

On the true meaning of the initials, WNL:
We never looked.
— *Anonymous* [94]

Medical definitions relating to the physical examination:
• Afebrile: Possessed of a body temperature between 0°F and 98.6°F.
• Deferred: Not done, and not likely to be done.
• Normocephalic: Head was present.
— *Faith T. Fitzgerald, MD* [127]

Dr. Wicksteed: The longer I practice medicine, the more convinced I am there are only two type of cases—those that involve taking the trousers off and those that don't.
— *Alan Bennett, "Habeas Corpus"* [31]

Dr. Wicksteed (chatting with a patient during an examination): It's all guess-work you know. I delve in their ears, I peer up their noses. I am glued to every orifice of the body like a parlor-maid at a keyhole.
— *Alan Bennett, "Habeas Corpus"* [31]

Crackles and rhonchi and sibilant wheezes,
Downgoing toes in a patient who seizes,
E. multiforme with concentric rings,
These are a few of my favorite things.
— *Howard Bennett, MD* [43]

A woman went to see a new doctor who turned out to be very handsome. He put his hand on her back and asked her to say "Ninety-nine."
    "Ninety-nine," she purred.
    Next, he put his hand on her throat and asked her to say "Ninety-nine" again.
    "Ninety-niiiiine," she said.
    "Fine," he said. "Now I'm going to put my hand on your chest and I want you to say 'Ninety-nine' one last time."
    "Okay," she said. "One, two, three, four . . ."

A doctor finished examining his patient and said, "I can't find a cause for your complaint, Mr. Jackson, but I think it's probably due to the drinking."
    "In that case," said the patient, "I'll come back when you're sober."

(See also Diagnosis, History & Physical Examination, Pelvic Exam, Prostate Gland, Rectal Exam, Stethoscope)

~ PIMPING ~

Pimping should do for the third-year student what the Senate hearings did for Robert Bork.
— *Frederick L. Brancati, MD* [63]

Clearly, pimping—good pimping—is an art. There are styles, approaches, and a few loose rules to guide the novice, but pimping is learned in practice, not theory.
— *Frederick L. Brancati, MD* [63]

Pimping, v. A popular form of entertainment in medical centers, occasionally interrupted by teaching.
— *Howard Bennett, MD* [46]

(See also Attendings, Roundsmanship)

~ PLACEBOS ~

If you must use placebos, for God's sake always make sure that those you use really do work!
— *Robert Matz, MD* [202]

If there was any justice in this world, HMO executives would always be in the placebo group.
— *Anonymous* [135]

Compared to Ben Casey, Dr. Kildare is a placebo.
— *Constance Rizzo* [258]

(See also Drugs)

~ PLASTIC SURGERY ~

She got her good looks from her father—he's a plastic surgeon.
— *Groucho Marx* [29]

We know more about the lifespan of automobile tires than we do about breast implants.
— *David Kessler, MD* [175]

I hear they can take the fat from your rear and use it to smooth out the dents in your face. Now, that's what I call recycling—it gives a whole new meaning to dancing cheek to cheek.
— *Anita Wise* [184]

What's the best way to make a million dollars?
— Become a plastic surgeon and work part-time.

How many plastic surgeons does it take to change a light bulb?
— Just one, but he'd prefer to reattach the old filament.

(See also Face Lifts, Liposuction, Nose Jobs)

~ PMDs ~

I don't think of myself as a PMD. I'm just academically challenged.
— *Rick Stevens, MD* [246]

In the event of a complication, always blame the PMD.
— *Anonymous* [94]

How many PMDs does it take to change a light bulb?
— Two. One to change the bulb and the other to double-bill the insurance company.

(See also Attendings)

~ PMS ~

Women complain about PMS, but I think of it as the only time of the month that I can be myself.
— *Roseanne Barr* [75]

The same time that women came up with PMS, men came up with ESPN.
— *Blake Clark* [76]

What's the difference between a woman with PMS and a terrorist?
— You can negotiate with a terrorist.

How many women with PMS does it take to change a light bulb?
— Six. Anybody have a problem with that?

(See also Menstruation)

~ PREGNANCY ~

My sister-in-law had a lot of gas when she was pregnant with her first child. One night was particularly eventful so I said, "Laura, would you mind going into another room until you're done?" She said, "If I left the room every time I had to pass gas, I'd never be here."
— *Howard Bennett, MD* [48]

When she's absolutely, positively sure she isn't pregnant, get a pregnancy test.
— *Oscar London, MD* [192]

After my first pregnancy, all of my fat went to my thighs. My husband's fat went to his head.
— *Molly Ryan, MD* [246]

If pregnancy were a book, they would cut the last two chapters.
— *Nora Ephron* [320]

How can I have morning sickness when I don't get up till noon?

— *Rita Rudner* [135]

The only time a women wishes she was a year older is when she's expecting a baby.

— *Mary Marsh* [247]

You know what they say when a supermodel gets pregnant? Now she's gonna be eating for one.

— *Jay Leno* [135]

I woke up with a start at 4:00 one morning and realized that I was very pregnant. Since I had conceived six months earlier, one might have thought that the news would have sunk in before then . . . What tipped me off was that, lying on my side and needing to turn over, I found myself unable to move. My first thought was that I had had a stroke.

— *Ann Lamott* [183]

Oh, what a tangled web we weave
When first we practice to conceive.

— *Don Herold* [191]

From a courtroom transcript:
Q: Do you know how pregnant you are right now?
A: I'll be four months on October 10th.
Q: So that means the date of conception was early June.
A: Yes.
Q: And what were you and your husband doing at the time?

A woman calls her insurance company to find out what her benefits are now that she is pregnant. Her agent says, "I'm sorry, Mrs. Wright, but your policy only pays for sickness and accidents."

"This was an accident," she answers.

A woman who is pregnant with her first child has a routine appointment with her obstetrician. When the visit is over, she shyly asks, "My husband wants me to ask you—"

"I know, I know," the doctor says. "People ask me that question all the time. You can do it as much as you want. It will be fine until late in the pregnancy."

Later that night, the woman's husband eagerly asks, "Well, what did the doctor say?"

The woman reassures her husband. "It'll be fine, honey. The doctor says I can still mow the lawn."

The doctor entered the waiting room. "I have some good news for you, Mrs. Davis."

"Pardon me," she interrupted, "but it's Miss."

"In that case, I have some bad news for you, Miss Davis."

A woman went to her doctor with a number of vague complaints. After examining the patient, the doctor said, "I'm not sure what this is, but it looks like you either have the flu or you're pregnant."

"Oh," the woman said. "Then I must be pregnant cause I don't know anyone who could have given me the flu."

A 60-year-old woman goes to the doctor and finds out, much to her surprise, that she is pregnant. She immediately calls her husband on the telephone. "You old coot," she says, "you got me pregnant."

The husband pauses for a moment, then says, "Who is this?"

What's the difference between worry and panic?
— About twenty-eight days.

(See also Biologic Clock, Childbirth, Obstetrics)

~ PRIMARY CARE ~

Rules of Primary Care:
• Patients always get better after they call for an appointment.
• Patients always develop the side effect you forgot to mention.
• If a spouse accompanies a patient, the visit will take twice as long.
• There's always a virus going around.
• Articles are never where you left them.
• Five o'clock patients are always late.
• Patients are never asleep when you stop by on rounds.
• If you get a blood test to reassure a patient, the results will always be abnormal.
• There are no interesting cases after midnight.
• Drug reps never get laryngitis.
• Minor complications only happen to other doctor's patients.
• Specialists never wait on hold.

An ad for a selling a general practice:
Solo practice located in a remote wilderness setting. Rugged townsfolk rarely get sick, though you will need to attend to livestock on occasion. Only 1200 miles from a major city, and no lawyers in the area.

(See also Medical Practice, PMDs)

~ PROCEDURES ~

I scope, therefore I am.

— *Anonymous* [94]

There is no body cavity that cannot be reached with a #14 needle and a good strong arm.

— *Samuel Shem, MD* [281]

When you don't know what you're doing, be real careful.

— *Ken Kuykendal, MD* [193]

Confidence is the feeling you have before you understand the situation.

— *Anonymous* [203]

The easy ones go across the street.

— *Richard L. Mabry, MD* [193]

If it looks easy, it's tough. If it looks tough, it's damn near impossible.

— *Anonymous* [201]

Allen's Law: Almost anything is easier to get into than out of. [203]

There are seven places in a man's body where nurses can stick a tube without making a new hole. I don't believe God ever intended for tubes to be stuck in several of those holes.

— *Lewis Grizzard* [148]

If a patient is doing well, don't just do something—Stand There!

— *Anonymous* [312]

Never try anything new on a Friday afternoon.

— *Anonymous* [94]

The more often you put your finger (or an instrument) in an orifice, the less often you will put your foot in your mouth.

— *Rip Pfeiffer, MD* [248]

See one, do one, miss one.

— *Anonymous* [94]

Dr. McCoy: Now this isn't going to hurt a bit.
Chekov: That's what you said last time.
Dr. McCoy: Did it hurt?
Chekov: Yes.

— *"Star Trek"* [284]

(See also Blood & Blood Drawing, Complications, Endoscopy, Informed Consent, IVs, Spinal Taps, Treatment)

~ PROCTOLOGY ~

A career in proctology is that rare profession in which the doctor starts at the bottom and stays there.

— *Anonymous* [135]

Rumor has it that the team of specialists who examined President Reagan's colon is known around Washington as the *Polypburo*.

— *Herb Caen* [77]

My father is a proctologist. My mother is an abstract artist. That's how I view the world.

— *Sandra Bernhardt* [163]

"We did that proctoscopy just in time," Dr. Palmer said. "In another 24 hours the patient would have gotten better without us."

A proctologist is about to write a report when he pulls a thermometer out of his pocket, looks at it and says, "Oh, damn, some asshole has my pen."

A proctologist is examining a patient when he asks his nurse for a light. She hands him a beer. "No," he says, "I mean a butt light."

As a young man, the British poet Alfred, Lord Tennyson was afflicted with a painful case of hemorrhoids. Accepting the recommendation of friends, he sought the advice of a young but well-known proctologist. The treatment was successful and for many years, Tennyson had no further trouble.

After he became famous, however, the poet suffered another attack. On visiting the proctologist, Tennyson expected to be recognized as the former patient who had become the great poet. The proctologist, however, gave no signs of recognition.

It was only when the noble lord bent over for his examination that the proctologist exclaimed, "Ah, Tennyson." [63]

Dr. Krauss performed a delicate eye operation and restored the vision of a famous painter. As a gesture of thanks, the artist presented Dr. Krauss with a portrait of the ophthalmologist inside a giant eyeball.

Dr. Krauss brought the painting home and showed it to his wife. "What do you think?" he asked.

After looking at it for a long time his wife said, "I'm glad I didn't marry a proctologist."

(See also Colonoscopy, Hemorrhoids)

~ PROSTATE GLAND ~

On prostate exams:
Most men survive the exam itself, even making jokes about it with their friends afterward. Some pretend they have endured some incredibly macho ordeal, like skydiving into an active volcano, which naturally makes their friends want to have theirs checked too. — *Mark DePaolis, MD* [108]

An old man from Denver named Lee
Had a prostate as big as a tree.
    Because of his plight,
    His sphincter was tight,
And it took him two hours to pee.
    — *Howard Bennett, MD* [48]

An 80-year-old man who was having some prostate trouble, asked his doctor to explain the function of his enigmatic gland.

"Well," said the doctor. "At your age, it's primary function is to make money for urologists like me."

(See also Rectal Exams, Urology)

~ PSYCHIATRY ~

A psychiatrist is the first person you talk to after you start talking to yourself.

— *Fred Allen* [135]

The first thing to do at a psychiatric emergency is to check your own mental status.

— *Samuel Shem, MD* [282]

Couches have been a part of psychiatrist's offices ever since Freud. He believed his patients would feel freer to talk when lying down, even though medical research clearly shows that most people who are lying down are either asleep or dead.

— *Mark DePaolis, MD* [108]

I told my mother that I was thinking about seeing a therapist. She thought that was a good idea because she heard they make a lot of money. — *Darlene Hunt* [67]

A psychiatrist is a Jewish doctor who can't stand the sight of blood.

— *Anonymous* [269]

Why is it that with psychiatrists every hour is only fifty minutes? What do they do with that ten minutes they have left? Do they just sit there going, "Boy that guy was crazy. I couldn't believe the things he was saying. What a nut. Who's coming in next? Oh no, another nut case."

— *Jerry Seinfeld* [275]

I'm so wracked with guilt. I don't want to stop therapy because I'm afraid to take the income away from my therapist. He's got kids in college.

— *Tim Halpern* [163]

How to be a good psychiatrist: Look smart, say nothing, and mumble a lot in German. — *Theodore Saretsky, Ph.D.* [273]

Show me a sane man and I will cure him for you. — *Carl Jung* [103]

Anybody who goes to a psychiatrist ought to have his head examined. — *Samuel Goldwyn* [283]

The superego is that part of the personality that is soluble in alcohol. — *Harold Lasswell, PhD* [247]

I don't trust any doctor who has a couch in his office. — *Larry Bauer, MD* [246]

Everybody knows that doctors make lousy patients. Psychiatrists are the worst. One of my psychiatrist dads called me last week to ask why his 5-year-old still had a fever on the third day of a cold. He put her on amoxicillin and was puzzled that she wasn't any better.

I said, "Look, Jim, I don't put my kids on Prozac just because they're in a bad mood." — *Rick Stevens, MD* [246]

Psychiatric Definitions:
• Fun: acting out
• Being late: passive aggressive
• Being early: passive dependent
• Being on time: compulsive
• Bad memory: resistance
• Daydreams (patient's): fantasies
• Daydreams (physician's): plans — *Charles T. Rumble, MD* [272]

Bloopers & Malapropisms:
• This patient has been under many psychiatrists in the past.
• This 48-year-old white female was referred by a local medical doctor who has a long psychiatric history.
• "My wife has had stomachaches for the past six months, but I think they're *psychoceramic.* (pschosomatic)

How can you tell the patients from the psychiatrists on a psych ward?
— The patients get better.

Hello and Welcome to the Psychiatric Hotline:
- If you are obsessive-compulsive, press 1 repeatedly.
- If you are co-dependent, ask someone to press 2 for you.
- If you have multiple personalities, press 3, 4, 5, and 6.
- If you are paranoid, we know who you are and what you do. Just stay on the line while we trace the call.
- If you are schizophrenic, listen carefully and a little voice will tell you which number to press.
- If you are depressed, it doesn't matter which number you press. No one will answer.
- If you are phobic, don't touch any buttons—something terrible will happen to you.
- If you are a narcissist, touch yourself.

Julie had been seeing a female therapist for eight years. One day her doctor suggested they terminate treatment saying, "You really don't need me anymore."

Three days later, Julie made a frantic call. "Dr. Samuels," she said, "you're like a mother to me. I just can't get through the day without you."

"Don't be silly," the therapist replied. "I'm not your mother, and you can make perfectly good decisions without me. Where are you now?"

"At home, eating breakfast."

"Good. And what are you having?"

"A cup of coffee."

"You call that breakfast?"

Two psychiatrists met on the street one day. The younger doctor says, "George, I don't know how you do it. How can you look so fresh after listening to patients complain day in and day out for all these years?"

The elder psychiatrist replies, "Who listens?"

"It was just awful," the man told his psychiatrist. "I was in San Francisco on business, and I wired my wife that I'd be back a day early. I rushed home from the airport and found her in bed with my best friend. I don't get it. How could she do this to me?"

"Well," said the psychiatrist after a long pause, "maybe she didn't get your telegram."

Two women are having lunch at a downtown restaurant. One of them says, "I've tried to get my husband into therapy for years, but he never goes."

"Why not?" her friend asks.

"He says what's the point in having an unconscious if you don't use it?"

"Everybody hates me," the patient said to his psychiatrist. "Don't be silly," the therapist replied. "Everybody hasn't met you yet."

How many psychiatric social workers does it take to change a light bulb?
— Five. One to screw it in and four to talk about how much they'll miss the old bulb.

(See also Anxiety, Depression, Family, Insanity, Multiple Personality Disorder, Obsessive-Compulsive Behavior, Personality Disorders, Phobias, Schizophrenia, Suicide)

~ PSYCHOANALYSIS ~

After being in suspended animation for 200 years, Woody Allen's character awakes in the movie *Sleeper* and says, "If I hadn't been asleep, I would almost be through with my analysis by now." [5]

Freud is the father of psychoanalysis. It had no mother.   — *Germaine Greer* [147]

It's weird that I have a parent who's a shrink. It's hard to think of my mom solving other people's problems when she's the root of all mine.
                                                              — *Carol Leifer* [163]

I was in analysis. I was suicidal. I would have killed myself but my analyst was a strict Freudian and if you kill yourself they make you pay for the sessions you miss.   — *Woody Allen* [194]

Psychoanalysis is spending $40 an hour to squeal on your mother.
                                                              — *Mike Connolly* [197]

My psychoanalyst used to be a teacher. If I show up late for a session, he makes me stand.

How many psychoanalysts does it take to change a light bulb?
— How many do you think it takes?

(See also Freud)

~ Psychology ~

Behavioral psychology is the science of pulling habits out of rats.

— Douglas Busch, PhD [247]

A few months ago, I read a study in a psychology journal about the behavior of men in public bathrooms. It turns out that it takes the average man 8 seconds to pee after he stands in front of a urinal. However, if another man comes into the bathroom, it takes an extra 5 seconds before the man begins to go. In fact, the closer anyone comes to this *average* man, the longer it takes for him to do his business. Now, *that* was a study that needed to be done.

— Larry Bauer, MD [246]

Any problem worth curing can be discussed in 50 minute blocks of time.

— Lawrence G. Calhoun, PhD et al. [80]

TV Interviewer: You mean you ask forty dollars an hour and you guarantee nothing?
Dr. Harley: Well, I validate.

— "The Bob Newhart Show" [57]

Object relations theories are derived from the supposition that "objects who need objects are the luckiest objects in the world." *— Carolyn Murphy, M.A.* [226]

A psychologist told a colleague, "Half of my patients come to me because they're married and the other half because they're not."

(See also Anxiety, Behavior Management, Neurotics)

~ Pulmonary Medicine ~

(See Lungs)

Q

~ QUACKS ~

Traditional medicine has not found an answer for your problem. However, luckily for you, I happen to be a quack.
— *Charles Richter* [74]

After successfully healing a woman who had been plagued by kidney disease all her life, Brother Roy Dodd bowed before his adoring audience. Suddenly, the woman fell off the stage and broke one of her legs. Several men in the audience rushed to her side. One suggested an ambulance, but another said, "We don't need an ambulance, we have Brother Dodd." Brother Roy stepped back and said, "I think you'd better call the ambulance. I don't do broken bones, just internal organs."
— *Lewis Grizzard* [148]

Edward Jenner sent the following epigram, along with a couple of ducks, to a patient:
    I've dispatched, my dear Madam, this scrap of a letter
    To say that Miss X is very much better;
    A regular doctor no longer she lacks,
    And therefore I've sent her a couple of quacks. [99]

Ross was sitting on the exam table in a well-known neurologist's office.
    "Tell me," the neurologist said, "did you see anyone else before coming to me for this problem?"
    "Yes," Ross said, "I saw my GP, Dr. Packer, last week."
    "That quack!" the neurologist said. "And what advice did *he* give you?"
    "He told me to come see you."

How many quacks does it take to change a light bulb?
—Just one, but it only works if the old bulb isn't really dead.

~ RADIOLOGY ~

Surgeons do it. Internists talk about it. Radiologists just like to look at the pictures.
— *Anonymous* [94]

From an actual chest x-ray report:
There is a faint suggestion of a wisp of density in the left retrocardiac area raising the question of a minimal pneumonia but equivocal at best.
— *Anonymous* [135]

My kids love to play doctor. Just last week, my 6-year-old examined one of his friends who had a stomachache. Ryan told Peter he needed a CAT scan, but Peter's big sister said their HMO wouldn't approve it without a second opinion. Ryan said he'd been a specialist for a zillion years and he'd be damned if some insurance company would question his clinical judgment. He said if Peter couldn't get the scan he wasn't playing anymore. So he came home and took a nap.
— *Howard Bennett, MD* [48]

If the radiology resident and the BMS (Best Medical Student) both see a lesion on the chest x-ray, there can be no lesion there. — *Samuel Shem, MD* [281]

Getting an x-ray done before noon in a teaching hospital is as likely as making it through attending rounds without being pimped. — *Howard Bennett, MD* [40]

Radiology Definitions:
• Barium: What you do to a patient if surgery fails.
• Cystogram: A wire sent to your sister.
• Isodense: What a med student says after taking the National Boards.
• Pleural: More than one.
• Sacral: Holy.
• Sella: A good place to keep wine.

Bloopers & Malapropisms:
- The chest x-ray reveals a density in the right lower lobe and a small pleural *allusion*. (effusion)
- The pelvic x-rays on this 25-year-old woman are *sensually* normal. (essentially)
- The patient was treated in the emergency room, *X-rated*, and released. (x-rayed)

Four doctors went duck hunting—an internist, a radiologist, a surgeon, and a pathologist. As they crouched in the grass, they agreed to let the internist shoot first. The first flock of birds approached and the internist raised his shotgun toward the sky. With a puzzled look on his face, he lowered his gun, only to raise it again as the ducks flew off. When his colleagues inquired why he didn't shoot, the internist replied, "When they were coming toward me, they looked like ducks. Then I looked again and thought they were geese. By the time I was sure they were ducks, they were gone." Next up was the radiologist. As the ducks flew towards the hunters, the barrel was raised and once again it was lowered. As the birds flew away the radiologist shook his head in frustration. "They looked like ducks in the lateral view, but I couldn't be sure until I saw the PA view. By then, they were gone." Next up was the surgeon. As the birds approached, he began firing wildly in all directions. Ducks fell from the sky like rain. When the smoke cleared, the surgeon gathered up all of the fallen fowl and handed them to the pathologist. "Here," he said triumphantly, "let me know if these are ducks or not?"

How do you hide a $100 bill from a radiologist?
— Stick it on a patient.

What's the leading cause of death among radiologists?
— Getting run over in the hospital parking lot at 3 PM by pathologists.

How many radiologists does it take to change a light bulb?
— Ten. One to screw it in and nine to sit around discussing the differential diagnosis of dead light bulbs.

(See also CAT Scans, Mammograms, X-Rays)

~ Rectal Examination ~

The rectal exam is that part of the physical examination that illustrates the true meaning of the Yuletide maxim, "It is better to give than to receive."

— *Howard Bennett, MD* [48]

On comparing rectal and pelvic exams:
Women have been having things like this done every year with very little whining, which is just another reason to be glad they are the ones giving birth. Given the choice, many men would simply say, "I hate this part," and the human species would never reproduce.

— *Mark DePaolis, MD* [108]

(See also Physical Diagnosis, Prostate Gland)

~ Research ~

To copy from one book is plagiarism; to copy from three is research.

— *Anonymous* [94]

There is no subject, however complex, which if studied with patience and intelligence, will not become more complex.

— *Robert Matz, MD* [201]

Don't count your subjects until they're batched.

— *Howard Bennett, MD* [40]

A drug is a substance that when injected into a guinea pig produces a scientific paper.

— *Anonymous* [94]

Get the facts first. You can distort them later.

— *Mark Twain* [19]

Gordon's Law: If a research project is not worth doing at all, it is not worth doing well. [201]

There is a need for two innovations that will round out the institutional framework of research—*The Fund for Dubious Projects* and *The Journal of Rejected Manuscripts*.

— *Daniel S. Greenberg* [146]

Researchers have already cast much darkness on this subject and if they continue their investigations we shall soon know nothing at all about it. — *Mark Twain* [194]

Medical research is advancing at an amazing rate. Every month the medical journals are full of reports like, "Blond, fair-skinned, left-handed pipe welders shown more susceptible to gallbladder disease . . ." — *Mark DePaolis, MD* [108]

Muench's Second Law: Results can always be improved by omitting controls. [202]

On triple blind studies:
The patients don't know what they're getting, the doctors don't know what they're giving, and no one knows what they're doing. — *Howard Bennett, MD* [34]

The hardest part of putting together a clinical trial is coming up with a catchy acronym for it. — *Daniel J. Waters, DO* [310]

Ambiguous questions lead inevitably to ambiguous results or, as computer scientists like to state, "garbage in, garbage out." — *Robert Matz, MD* [201]

Cardiologists believe that experiments in dogs are essential, but antivivisectionists oppose research in animals. There is a solution to this dilemma—use lawyers instead of dogs. The one problem, of course, is extrapolating the results from lawyers to humans. — *Charles Hennekens, MD* [155]

Money won't buy happiness, but it will pay the salaries of a large research staff to study the problem. — *Bill Vaughn* [12]

Why have laboratories switched from rats to lawyers in their experiments?
• There's no shortage of lawyers.
• You don't get attached to them.
• There are some things even rats won't do.

How many researchers does it take to change a light bulb?
— Three. One to write the grant proposal, one to design a $250 bulb, and one to train the lab tech to put it in.

(See also Grants, Statistics, Tenure, Writing & Publishing)

~ RESIDENCY ~

(See Internship & Residency)

~ RETIREMENT ~

A doctor is happiest twice in his life—the day he hangs his diploma up and the day he takes it down.
— *Howard Bennett, MD* [40]

How many retired docs does it take to change a light bulb?
— Three. One to screw it in and two to reminisce about how much easier it was to change bulbs in the old days.

~ RHEUMATOLOGY ~

The best medicine I know for rheumatism is to thank the Lord it ain't the gout.
— *Josh Billings* [125]

Two women were waiting to see their rheumatologist when they got to talking about their respective ailments. "I can't wait to try that new pain medicine that everyone's talking about," one of them said.

"I agree," said the other woman. "I hear it works like aspirin, but costs much more."

How many rheumatologists does it take to change a light bulb?
— None. That's what fellows are for.

(See also Arthritis, Gout, Knees, Lyme Disease)

~ ROUNDSMANSHIP ~

The most important sign is the one no one else has found.   — *Ian Rose, MD* [264]

There is no human being whose medical characteristics cannot be listed on a three-by-five card. *— Samuel Shem, MD* (281)

When in trouble, mumble. *— Leo Rosten* (268)

The longer a patient is discussed on rounds, the more certain it is that no one has the faintest idea what's going on or what to do. *— Alan Spitzer, MD* (292)

With sombre mien, with chin on chest,
Thumbs in the pockets of the vest,
Attendings study learning's voids
And contemplate their hemorrhoids. *— Samuel P. Bessman, MD* (50)

On being grilled during hospital rounds:
The incidence of anything worthwhile is either 15–25 percent or 80–90 percent.
— Michael A. LaCombe, MD (182)

No matter how well you have examined your patients, the attending physician will always want to see the one you didn't have time to get around to.
— Robert J. Joynt, MD (170)

If you can't dazzle them with brilliance, baffle them with data. *— Anonymous* (94)

Stat, v. An indication that someone forgot to order a test before rounds.
— Anonymous (94)

It is better to keep your mouth shut and appear stupid than to open it and remove all doubt. *— Mark Twain (attrib.)* (283)

An ounce of pretension is worth a pound of manure. *— Steven E. Clark* (92)

Famous lines said on rounds:
• Results are pending.
• The computer is down.
• The specimen was lost.

- My beeper was dead.
- The patient was in radiology when I went to check him.
- My alarm didn't go off.
- No one paged me.
- The patient doesn't speak English.
- The old chart is missing.
- The patient didn't tell me that.

(See also Case Presentations, Diagnosis, Pearls, Pimping, PMDs, Turfing)

S

~ SCARS ~

A sexy young woman had surgery for an inguinal hernia. After the operation, her surgeon stopped by to see how she was doing. "I'm doing very well, Dr. Hartman, but I was wondering if the scar will show?"

"My dear," replied the doctor, "that is entirely up to you."

~ SCIENCE & SCIENTISTS ~

It is inexcusable for scientists to torture animals; let them make their experiments on journalists and politicians. — *Henrik Ibsen* [168]

Phinagle's Credo: Science is truth. Don't be misled by the facts. [216]

Science is a wonderful thing if one does not have to earn one's living at it. — *Albert Einstein* [118]

Two leading Congressional scientists, Senator Helms and Representative Hyde, have been doing pioneering research on the nature of life. This has produced the Helms-Hyde theory which states that scientific fact can be established by a majority vote of the United States Congress. — *Russel Baker* [21]

Alexander Fleming was once asked by a journalist what a great scientist thinks about when he sits down to breakfast.

"It's curious you should ask me that," Fleming replied. "It so happens that I am thinking about something rather special."

"What is it?" the journalist asked excitedly.

"Well," Fleming said, "I was wondering whether I should have one egg or two." [99]

(See also Research)

~ Schizophrenia ~

You don't have to be a schizophrenic to treat a schizophrenic. — *Anonymous* [94]

Schizophrenia beats dining alone. — *Oscar Levant* [186]

A young schizophrenic named Struther,
When told of the death of his brother,
   Said, "Yes, it's too bad,
   But I can't feel too sad—
After all, I still have each other." — *Anonymous* [241]

(See also Insanity, Psychiatry)

~ Scut ~

Scut, n. Chores that have hypertrophied. — *Howard Bennett, MD* [46]

There are many advantages to being a resident, but chief among them is that now I get to make out the scut list. — *Molly Ryan, MD* [246]

There once was a student named Tutt,
Who spent his whole day doing scut.
   "I take bloods to the lab,
   Never stopping to gab,
While my intern's upstairs on his butt." — *Howard Bennett, MD* [48]

(See also Pearls)

~ Second Opinions ~

Getting a second doctor's opinion is like switching slot machines.
— *Jimmy Townsend* [135]

Telling someone he looks healthy isn't a compliment—it's a second opinion.

— *Fran Lebowitz* [135]

A woman with abdominal pain goes to see the doctor. After a brief examination, the doctor tells her she has inflamed gallstones and needs an operation right away. The woman decides to get another opinion. The second doctor tells her she has indigestion and heart trouble. "I'm going back to the first doctor," the woman says. "I'd rather have gallstones."

Three college roommates got together regularly over the years even though their professional lives took them in different directions. One had become a biologist, one an architect, and the third, a businessman.

At their latest meeting, all three men were depressed because it turned out that each had been told by his doctor that he only had two months to live. Understandably, the conversation turned to the way each man intended to live out his last days.

"I'm going to Africa," said the biologist. "I've always wanted to see the rare mountain gorilla in its native habitat."

"Greece for me," said the architect. "What a treat it will be to spend my final days where civilization began."

"And you?" asked the biologist, turning to the third friend. "What would you like to see?"

The businessman paused for a moment and said, "Another doctor."

A doctor and his wife have a big fight during breakfast. After arguing for thirty minutes, the husband shouts, "You aren't so good in bed either," and storms off to work. By lunchtime, he's feeling pretty guilty and decides to call his wife to apologize. After many rings, his wife picks up the phone.

"What took you so long to answer?" the doctor asks.

"I was in bed."

"What were you doing in bed this late?"

"Getting a second opinion."

(See also Advice)

~ SELF HELP ~

I've bought a lot of self-help books over the years, but they never seem to help. Apparently, you have to read them.

— *Ryan James, MD* [246]

THE DOCTOR'S BOOK OF HUMOROUS QUOTATIONS / 231

I went into a bookstore and asked the woman behind the counter where the self-help section was. She said, "If I told you that, it would defeat the whole purpose."

— *Brian Kiley* [135]

I have a new book coming out. It's one of those self-help deals. It's called "How to Get Along with Everyone." I wrote it with this other jerk.   — *Steve Martin* [307]

In the year 2000, authors of self-help books will be required to provide proof that they have actually helped themselves.

— *Jane Wagner* [307]

There are a lot of self-help tapes out there. I got one called, "How to Handle Disappointment." I took it home and the box was empty.   — *Jonathan Droll* [186]

I was going to buy a copy of *The Power of Positive Thinking*, and then I thought, "What the hell good would that do?"

— *Ronnie Shakes* [96]

The problem with self-improvement is knowing when to quit.

— *David Lee Roth* [186]

(See also Health Care Books)

~ SEX ~

Mrs. Harvey, your stitches will come out in seven or eight days so there is no reason why in about two weeks you cannot begin denying your husband sex again.

— *Mark Bryant* [194]

New research shows that the more sex a man has, the more he wants. Not only that, the research also shows the less sex a man has, the more he wants.

— *Conan O'Brien* [135]

Sex therapists think the whole problem is that we don't communicate enough. Dr. Ruth says as women we should *tell* our partners how to make love to us. My boyfriend goes nuts if I tell him how to *drive*.   — *Pam Stone* [195]

I have low self-esteem. When we were in bed together, I would fantasize that I was someone else. — *Richard Lewis* [84]

Sex when you're married is like going to a 7-Eleven. There's not much variety, but at three in the morning, it's always there. — *Carol Leifer* [84]

Sonja: Sex without love is an empty experience.
Boris: Yes, but as empty experiences go, it's one of the best.
— *Woody Allen, "Love & Death"* [6]

According to old Sigmund Freud,
Life is seldom so well enjoyed
   As in human coition,
   In any position,
With the usual organs employed. — *Anonymous* [241]

Women need a reason to have sex. Men just need a place.
— *Billy Crystal, "City Slickers"* [90]

Luna: Do you want to perform sex with me?
Miles: Perform sex? I don't think I'm up to a performance, but I'll rehearse with you if you'd like. — *Woody Allen, "Sleeper"* [5]

The enjoyment of sex, although great,
Is in later years said to abate.
   This well may be so,
   But how would I know?
I'm now only seventy-eight. — *Anonymous* [241]

Remember when "Safe Sex" meant your parents had gone away for the week-end? — *Rhonda Hansome* [196]

I'm at the in between age—I still want sex badly, I just want it before 10 PM.
— *Kim Castle* [67]

If sex is such a natural phenomenon, how come there are so many books on how to? — *Bette Midler* [103]

It's hard for me to get used to these changing times. I can remember when the air was clean and sex was dirty. — *George Burns* [96]

Said a pretty young student named Smith,
Whose virtue was largely a myth,
  "Try hard as I can
  I can't find a man
Who it's fun to be virtuous with." — *Anonymous* [308]

Sex drive is a physical craving that begins in adolescence and ends at marriage. — *Robert Byrne* [196]

Male sexual response is far brisker and more automatic—it is triggered easily by things, like putting a quarter in a vending machine. — *Alex Comfort* [62]

"I'm eighty years old, but I can only have sex once a month," George Burns said to his doctor.
  "That's normal," his doc said.
  "Maybe so," Burns complained, "but Groucho Marx is eighty-five and he says he has sex twice a week."
  "Okay," replied the doctor, "you say the same thing."

An old man went to see his doctor for a checkup. At the end of the visit the doctor said, "I think you should cut your sex life in half."
  "Which half," the man said, "talking about it or thinking about it?"

A third year medical student was taking a long time with his first history and physical examination. Forty-five minutes into the interview, he got around to asking the patient if she was sexually active. She answered, "I might be if you'd hurry up and finish."

The night before her wedding, Holly pulled her mother aside for an intimate little chat. "Mom," she confided, "I want you to tell me how I can make my new husband happy."
  The bride's mother took a deep breath, "Well, Holly," she began, "when two people love and respect each other, sex can be a beautiful thing."
  "Mom, I know how to make love," interrupted the girl. "What I want you to do is teach me how to make lasagna."

What's the difference between anxiety and panic?

— Anxiety is the first time you can't do it a second time. Panic is the second time you can't do it the first time.

A woman goes to her doctor complaining that she is tired all of the time. After the diagnostic tests show nothing, the doctor asks her how often she has intercourse.

"Every Monday, Wednesday, and Saturday," she says.

The doctor advises her to cut out Wednesdays.

"I can't," the woman says. "That's the only night I'm home with my husband."

Randy Plotkin, a world-renowned urologist and expert on sexual dysfunction, was asked by a women's group to give a lecture on his specialty. Giving his standard talk about sex was an easy request to fill, but he decided to give a lecture on sailing instead.

The doctor knew very little about sailing, but promised himself to take time out from his busy schedule to learn about the sport. He went to the library to read about sailing and borrowed videotapes on sailing races. But when he arrived at the auditorium to give his talk, Plotkin felt a moment of panic about lecturing on a subject he still knew very little about. So instead, he gave his usual talk about sexual intercourse. The women were thrilled and applauded him wildly.

That afternoon, one of the women in the audience ran into the doctor's wife and gushed about what a wonderful speech he had given. "You must be very proud, Mrs. Plotkin. Your husband is such a good speaker and is so knowledgeable about his subject."

Mrs. Plotkin was taken aback. "Knowledgeable? He's only done it twice. Once he got sick and the other time his hat blew off!"

An older man was married to a younger woman. After five years of a very happy marriage, he had a heart attack. The doctor advised him that to prolong his life he needed to cut out the sex.

The man and his wife discussed the problem and decided that he would sleep in the family room downstairs to save them both from temptation.

One night, several weeks later, he decided that life without sex wasn't worth living, so he headed upstairs. He met his wife on the staircase and said, "I was coming up to die."

She laughed and replied, "I was coming down to kill you."

(See also Marriage, Masturbation, Penis, Vagina)

~ Sex Education ~

People want sex education out of the schools. They believe sex education causes promiscuity. Hey, I took algebra, but I never do math.   — *Elayne Boosler* [163]

Telling a teenager the facts of life is like giving a fish a bath.   — *Arnold Glasow* [105]

They say teaching sex education in the public schools will promote promiscuity. With our educational system? If we promote promiscuity the same way we promote math or science, they've got nothing to worry about.   — *Beverly Mickins* [135]

Advice on sex to young students:
Be abstinent, but under protest.   — *Sigmund Freud* [99]

(See also Birth Control, Condoms)

~ Sexually Transmitted Disease ~

(See Venereal Disease)

~ Sleep ~

The amount of sleep required by the average person is just five minutes more.
— *Anonymous* [103]

The definition of adulthood is that you want to sleep.   — *Paula Poundstone* [203]

We're pretty strict about sleep habits in my house. The only thing that's allowed to wake me up at 5 AM is my bladder.   — *Howard Bennett, MD* [48]

I don't mind sleeping on an empty stomach provided it isn't mine.
— *Philip J. Simborg* [75]

Man is the only animal that goes to bed when he's not sleepy and gets up when he is. — *Anonymous* [218]

If we can develop some way in which a man can doze (in public) and still keep from making a monkey of himself, we have removed one of the big obstacles to human happiness in modern civilization. — *Robert Benchley* [116]

The average, healthy, well-adjusted adult gets up at 7:30 in the morning feeling just plain terrible. — *Jean Kerr* [103]

When I woke up this morning my girlfriend asked me, "Did you sleep good?" I said, "No, I make a few mistakes." — *Steven Wright* [135]

People who say they sleep like a baby usually don't have one. — *Leo J. Burke* [247]

Early to rise and early to bed makes a male healthy and wealthy and dead. — *James Thurber* [103]

(See also Insomnia, Snoring)

~ SMOKING ~

It is now proven, beyond a doubt, that smoking is a leading cause of statistics. — *Fletcher Knebel* [103]

People are so rude to smokers. You'd think they'd try to be nicer to people that are dying. — *Roseanne Barr* [242]

"Light" cigarettes are no safer than any other brand; smoking light cigarettes to stay healthy is like using only low-caliber ammunition to shoot yourself. — *Mark DePaolis, MD* [108]

To cease smoking is the easiest thing I ever did. I ought to know because I've done it a thousand times. — *Mark Twain* [19]

The most common reason that people stop smoking in death.

— Mark DePaolis, MD [110]

Those nicotine patches seem to work pretty well, but I understand it's hard to keep 'em lit.

— George Carlin [186]

The Surgeon General has determined that the only smokers who don't inhale are dead smokers.

— Oscar London, MD [192]

I quit smoking. I feel better. I smell better. And it's safer to drink out of old beer cans laying around the house.

— Roseanne Barr [163]

The stigma of being fat is nothing compared to that of being a smoker. If a fat person eats a double burrito, that burrito is history. There is no talk about second-hand cholesterol from the refried beans causing heart disease among passers-by.

— Michael Robertson [259]

I smoke cigars because at my age, if I don't have something to hold onto, I might fall down.

— George Burns [135]

A woman said to me, "Is it true that you still go out with young girls?" I said, "Yes, it's true." She said, "It is true that you still smoke 15 cigars a day?" I said, "Yes, it's true." She said, "It is true that you still take a few drinks a day?" I said, "Yes, it's true." She said, "What does your doctor say?" I said, "He's dead."

— George Burns [106]

~ SNEEZING ~

(See Allergy)

~ SNORING ~

There's only one sure cure for snoring—insomnia.

— Gene Perret [244]

Laugh and the world laughs with you; snore and you sleep alone.

— Anthony Burgess [125]

(See also Sleep)

~ SORE THROAT ~

(See Strep Throat)

~ SPECIALISTS ~

A specialist is someone who learns more and more about less and less until he knows everything about nothing. A generalist is someone who learns less and less about more and more until he knows nothing about everything.

— Anonymous [94]

A specialist is a doctor with a smaller practice but a bigger boat.

— Tom Charlton [29]

An expert doesn't know any more than you do. He's just better organized and uses slides.

— Stephen Brunton, MD [70]

When a specialist says, "After an exhaustive work-up, a review of the literature, and a discussion with my colleagues, we have not yet arrived at a definitive diagnosis for your patient," what he really means is, "Damned if I know what's going on."

— Howard Bennett, MD [37]

The specialist must always appear to be fond of the general practitioner in the same way a good citizen in fond of his dog or the Mountie is fond of his horse.

— Ian Rose, MD [264]

The month you're on service always has three times as many days as any other month in the year.

— Alan Spitzer, MD [292]

It's a bad sign when the number of specialists on a case is greater than the number of members in the patient's family. — *Anonymous* [135]

General practitioners are never right but may, on occasion, not be wrong. — *Ian Rose, MD* [264]

Specialists suffer from two problems—First, their patients think they know everything. And second, so does the specialist. — *Graeme Garden, MD* [137]

The only way to get the same opinion from a group of three specialists is if two of them are on vacation. — *Howard Bennett, MD* [40]

In this age of specialization, what four out of five doctors end up recommending is another doctor. — *Jeff Rovin* [186]

The problem with calling in a consultant is that you may feel obligated to take his advice. — *Robert Matz, MD* [201]

A specialist is someone who never met a procedure he didn't like. — *Ryan James, MD* [246]

What's the definition of a consultant?
— Someone who can tell you a thousand ways to make love, but doesn't know any woman.

Bobby Miller was a retired baseball player who was down on his luck and in need of an operation. He asked around and was referred to the most respected and expensive specialist in town.

"Doc, I've been told that I need this expensive operation," Miller explained.

"You're right," the doctor replied. "You do need the procedure, and it costs $20,000 to perform."

"C'mon, doc, times are tough. I didn't make the big bucks when I played ball so I can't afford that much."

"I'll tell you what I'll do," the doctor responded. "I used to be a big fan of yours, so I'll do it for $2,000 and one of your old uniforms."

"That's still too steep," the old ballplayer replied.

They haggled back and forth, and finally settled on $100 and a baseball cap the old timer wore in his last World Series.

As Miller got up to leave, the specialist said, "Tell me, if you knew I was the most expensive doctor in town, why did you come to me?"

"Heck, doc," replied Miller. "where my health is concerned, money is no object."

(See also Generalist, Second Opinions)

~ SPINAL TAPS ~

If it takes more than three people to hold a child down for a spinal tap, he probably doesn't need one.
— *Anonymous* [94]

During the course of a spinal tap, a patient will hear the six most commonly told lies in medicine:
• I've done this a million times.
• This won't hurt a bit.
• Here's a little bee sting.
• The worst is over now.
• We're almost done.
• Not that wasn't so bad was it?   — *George Thomas, MD & Lee Schreiner, MD* [303]

(See also Procedures)

~ SPINE ~

The spine is a series of bones running down your back. You sit on one end of it and your head sits on the other.
— *Anonymous* [125]

~ SPLEEN ~

When the spleen is found on the right side, the patient should consider switching physicians.
— *S. N. Gaño, MD* [136]

During a lecture on anemia, a hematology professor asked a medical student to outline the functions of the spleen. After a few minutes the anxious student replied, "I used to know, sir, but I've forgotten what they are." The professor answered, "Good Lord, now nobody knows." — *Graeme Garden, MD* [137]

~ Sports Medicine ~

I went skiing last week and broke a leg. Fortunately, it wasn't mine.
— *Anonymous* [217]

I won't participate in any sport that has ambulances at the bottom of the hill.
— *Erma Bombeck* [194]

(See also Orthopedics)

~ Statistics ~

Statistics will prove anything, even the truth. — *Lord Moynihan* [298]

The average human being has one breast and one testicle. — *Stephen Grollman* [194]

Statistics, n. A group of numbers looking for an argument. — *Anonymous* [71]

Never try to walk across a river just because it has an average depth of four feet.
— *Martin Friedman* [75]

A comment made in the acknowledgement section of a research paper:
Thanks to Dr. R. G. Newcombe for his expert statistical advice which, as usual, we partly followed. — *Alan Fraser, MD, et al.* [130]

Medical statistics are like a bikini. What they reveal is interesting, but what they conceal is vital. — *Anonymous* [298]

Statistics are like old medical journals or like revolvers in a newly opened mining district. Most men rarely use them and find it troublesome to preserve them for easy access. However, when they do want them, they want them badly.

— *John Shaw Billings* [53]

There are two kinds of statistics, the kind you look up and the kind you make up.

— *Rex Stout* [103]

There are three kinds of lies—lies, damned lies, and statistics.   — *Mark Twain* [19]

How many statisticians does it take to change a light bulb?
— One . . . plus or minus three.

(See also Research)

~ STETHOSCOPE ~

The most important part of the stethoscope is the part between the ears.

— *Anonymous* [94]

~ STREP THROAT ~

People with positive throat cultures never have phones.   — *Anonymous* [94]

An updated version of the above:
People with positive throat cultures always have cell phones—and they never work.

— *Rick Stevens, MD* [246]

If you treat a strep throat it lasts a week, and if you don't treat it, it lasts seven days.

— *Anonymous* [94]

~ STRESS ~

I read this article. It said the typical symptoms of stress are eating too much, smoking too much, impulse buying, and driving too fast. Are they kidding? This is my idea of a great day!
— *Monica Piper* [186]

Stress wasn't always a bad thing. In earlier times, stress was due to the very real possibility of being eaten by wolves. Our ancestors learned to respond with surges of adrenaline, which allowed them to face the oncoming wolves and, in a sudden burst of incredible strength, push other people into their path.
— *Mark DePaolis, MD* [108]

(See also Anxiety)

~ SUICIDE ~

You want to go easy on the suicide stuff—first thing you know, you'll ruin your health.
— *Robert Benchley* [116]

I was suicidal. As a matter of fact, I would have killed myself, but I was in analysis with a strict Freudian, and if you kill yourself they make you pay for the sessions you miss.
— *Woody Allen* [96]

Your health comes first; you can always hang yourself later.
— *Folk Saying* [135]

Mrs. Wicksteed (picking up the telephone): Dr. Wicksteed's residence. Oh, it's you Mr. Purdue. No, you cannot speak to Dr. Wicksteed, this is his afternoon off. You're about to commit suicide? I see. Well, if you must commit suicide on the doctor's afternoon off, that's your funeral.
— *Alan Bennett, "Habeas Corpus"* [31]

Allan Felix (trying to pick-up a girl): What are you doing Saturday night?
Girl in Museum: Committing suicide.
Allan: What about Friday night?
— *Woody Allen, "Play It Again Sam"* [4]

Patient: When I woke up this morning, I felt so bad I tried to kill myself by taking a whole bottle of Tylenol.
Doctor: Really? What happened?
Patient: After the first two, I felt better.

~ SUPEREGO ~

The superego is that part of the personality that is soluble in alcohol.

— *Harold Lasswell, Ph.D.* [247]

~ SURGEON GENERAL ~

I came here as prime steak and now I feel like low-grade hamburger.

— *Joyceln Elders, MD* [119]

Top Ten Surgeon General Pet Peeves:
1. Cabinet members are always asking for free medical advice.
2. Tobacco company CEOs no longer send you Christmas cards.
3. None of the toy companies make a Surgeon General action figure.
4. You can't use your beeper to get out of meetings anymore.
5. During confirmation hearings, someone always brings up that you never understood the Krebs cycle.
6. You're not allowed to experiment on guys who beat you up in high school.
7. You have to stay awake at State of the Union speeches.
8. Can't use Air Force One to get carryout from Bob's Famous Chicken 'n' Ribs.
9. People expect you to know the answers to all the medical questions on *Jeopardy*.
10. You have to wear a bathing suit in the president's hot tub.

— *Howard Bennett, MD* [42]

~ SURGEONS ~

An internist is someone who knows everything and does nothing. A surgeon is someone who knows nothing and does everything. A pathologist is someone who knows everything and does everything but too late. — *Anonymous* [94]

Never let the skin stand between you and the diagnosis. — *Anonymous* [94]

All my life, as a golfer, I have tried to lay them cold and stiff at the holeside, and as a surgeon I have always tried to do the opposite. — *Lord Moynihan* [99]

The number of supplies and instruments a surgeon says he'll need is inversely related to the amount he will ultimately require. — *Patty Swenson, RN* [300]

Never ask a surgeon if he thinks you need an operation. — *Anonymous* [248]

Surgeons do it. Internists talk about it. Radiologists just like to look at the pictures. — *Anonymous* [94]

A fashionable surgeon, like a pelican, can be recognized by the size of his bill.
— *J. Chalmers Da Costa, MD* [102]

On being taken to the operating room after being shot by James Hinkley:
I hope my surgeon is a Republican. — *Ronald Reagan* [193]

Said the resident surgeon, John Galium,
"When I take call I don't dilly-dally 'em.
　　I'm carving till dawn
　　With barely a yawn,
While the Chairman's in bed with his Valium." — *Rick Stevens, MD* [246]

The average surgeon's concept of time is the eighth wonder of the world—if a surgeon says, "This will only take 45 minutes," DOUBLE it!
— *Patty Swenson, RN* [300]

Our doctor would never really operate unless it was necessary. He was just that way. If he didn't need the money, he wouldn't lay a hand on you.
— *Herb Shriner* [103]

I dated a surgical resident last Thanksgiving. When we carved the turkey, he made me hold the retractor. — *Molly Ryan, MD* [246]

What do you call a surgeon who mistakenly operates on the wrong leg?
— A defendant.

A surgeon, an internist, and a family practitioner go duck hunting.

The surgeon sees a duck, shouts "Duck!" and shoots it down.

The internist sees a duck, shouts "Duck! Rule out quail! Rule out pheasant!" and shoots it down.

The family practitioner sees a duck and blasts it out of the sky with a burst of machine-gun fire. As the tattered carcass falls to the ground, he remarks "I don't know what the hell it was, but I sure got it."

(For a variation on this joke, see page 197.)

"I'm terrified," the patient said to her surgeon. "This is the first operation I've ever had."

"I know just how you feel," the surgeon said. "This is the first operation I've ever done."

How many surgeons does it take to change a light bulb?
—Two. One to change the bulb and the other to say, "I haven't seen anyone do that outdated procedure in years."

How can you hide $100 from a surgeon?
— Give it to his wife and kids.

How do you keep a secret from a surgeon?
— Publish it in a medical journal.

~ SURGERY ~

After surgery, patients are taken to the recovery room, where they begin the most important job they will have over the next few days—*not bleeding*.
— *Mark DePaolis, MD* [110]

There's nothing wrong with you that an expensive operation can't prolong.

— *Graham Chapman* [196]

These days they rarely use stitches to close wounds after surgery. Instead, they use staples, which are easier for the surgeon. This bothers some people, who would rather not have a major procedure where they put you back together using office supplies.

— *Mark DePaolis, MD* [110]

When you don't know what you're cutting, don't.

— *M.C. Culbertson, MD* [193]

Scissors, n. An instrument used by medical students to cut surgical knots too short or too long.

— *Howard Bennett, MD* [46]

I am sometimes asked to operate only on days when the stars are favorable to the patient. I readily accede to this—it helps to spread the responsibility.

— *A. Dickson Wright, MD* [99]

On the proper frame of mind before undergoing surgery:
Console yourself with the reflection that you are giving the doctor pleasure, and that he is getting paid for it.

— *Mark Twain* [19]

This is a hospital filled with a lot of doctors and nurses. When you have doctors and nurses, you have a lot of operating going on—some of it even in surgery.

— *Hawkeye Pierce, "M*A*S*H"* [200]

"Closed" is a relative term to a surgeon.

— *Richard Conti, MD* [97]

A minor operation is one performed on someone else.

— *Anonymous* [94]

There are no unnecessary operations, however, some are more necessary than others.

— *Rip Pfeiffer, MD* [248]

A chance to cut is a chance to cure.

— *Rip Pfeiffer, MD* [248]

The operation was successful, but the patient died.

— *Anonymous* [94]

Never operate on the wrong leg—especially if the patient is a lawyer.

— Ryan James, MD [246]

I cut, therefore I am.

— Anonymous [94]

Before undergoing a surgical operation, arrange your temporal affairs. You may live.

— Ambrose Bierce [51]

Never say "Oops!" in the operating room.

— Leo Troy, MD [322]

It was dry when we closed.

— Anonymous [216]

When in doubt, cut it out.

— Anonymous [94]

Bloopers & Malapropisms:
• The patient was seen in consultation by Dr. Ross who felt we should sit on the abdomen, and I agree.
• The patient has bilateral varicosities below the legs.
• On physical examination, the patient's *vowel* sounds were normal. (bowel)
• We had to put in a central line because of poor venous *axis*. (access)
• The patient had surgery for a *high anal* hernia. (hiatal)
• We closed the incision with *five old nylons*. (5-0 nylon)
• Ever since Mrs. Wilson had her gallbladder removed, she can't tolerate greasy *males*. (meals)
• The patient was scheduled to have a bowel resection. However, he took a job as a stockbroker instead.
• The patient was released to the outpatient department without dressing.
• The patient was guarded and had a *frigid* abdomen. (rigid)
• The patient consulted a vascular surgeon to see what could be done about her *very close* veins. (varicose)
• After exposing the gallbladder, we ligated the cystic *duck*. (duct)
• The hospital operator announced the start of Morbidity & *Morality* Rounds. (mortality)

How do you recognize a surgeon in the OR?
— He has blood stains on his clogs.

How do you recognize an anesthesiologist in the OR?
— He has coffee stains on his clogs.

Dr. Newman was attending a dinner party and watched as the host adroitly carved a large turkey for his guests.

"How am I doing, doc?" the host said. "I bet I'd make a pretty good surgeon."

When the host was through stacking the sliced turkey on the serving plate, the surgeon looked up and said, "Anybody can take 'em apart Harry. Now let's see you put it back together."

Mr. Kahn was somber as he entered the doctor's office.

"There's no doubt about it," said the surgeon, "you need this operation. But I must inform you that it's a dangerous procedure, and two out of three patients don't survive."

"I see," the patient said.

"But I wouldn't worry about it, Mr. Kahn. I know you'll make it."

"How can you be so sure?"

"Because my last two patients died."

(See also Anesthesia, Appendix, Gallbladder, Hemorrhoids, Hernia, Informed Consent, Morbidity & Mortality Conference, Pancreas, Procedures, Transplantation, Varicose Veins)

~ SYMPTOMS ~

You can't make an asymptomatic patient better.   — *Anonymous* [298]

$\mathcal{T}$

~ TEACHING ~

(See Education)

~ TEENAGERS ~

(See Adolescence)

~ TEETH ~

I've got a tooth that's driving me to extraction. — *Charlie McCarthy* [217]

Adam and Eve had many advantages, but the principal one was that they escaped teething. — *Mark Twain* [19]

On removing an impacted wisdom tooth:
If at first you don't succeed, pry, pry again. — *Anonymous* [135]

Nothing dentured, nothing gained. — *Dental Slogan* [135]

Said the mother whose babe had been teething,
"He was crying in bed, really seething.
　　But now he's asleep,
　　Not making a peep,
Should we wake him to make sure he's breathing?" — *Howard Bennett, MD* [41]

~ TENURE ~

Tenure is the status granted by a medical center that guarantees your employment until you die or they are purchased by a for-profit hospital chain, whichever comes first.
— *Howard Bennett, MD* [48]

Getting published is a drive that begins in residency and ends with tenure.
— *Howard Bennett, MD* [48]

Why God never got tenure at a university:
• He only had one major publication.
• It was in Hebrew.
• It had no references.
• It wasn't published in a refereed journal.
• There was no placebo group.
• He never applied to the Ethic's Board for permission to experiment on human subjects.
• The scientific community has been unable to replicate his results.
• It may be true that he created the world, but what has he done since then?
• He rarely came to class and just told his students to read The Book.
• His office hours were infrequent and usually held on a mountain top.

(See also Academia, Research, Writing & Publishing)

~ THUMB SUCKING ~

A young boy had the habit of sucking his thumb. His mother tried everything to get him to stop, but nothing worked. Finally, one day she pointed to a man with a very large belly and said, "Tommy, that man has a big stomach because he sucked his thumb as a child."

The next day the boy accompanied his mother to the supermarket, and he kept staring at a woman who was about eight months pregnant. The woman got a bit annoyed and said, "Please stop staring young man, you don't know me."

"No," said the boy, "but I know what you've been doing."

~ Toilet Training ~

A watched tot never soils.

— Howard Bennett, MD [48]

The baby is great. My wife and I just started potty training. Which is important, I think, because if we wanna potty train the baby, we should set an example.

— Howie Mandel [67]

~ Tonsils ~

(See Strep Throat)

~ Transplantation ~

On February 10, 1929, Karl Benz, inventor of the Mercedes-Benz died. Doctors might have saved him, but they couldn't get the parts.   *— Marty Cohen* [95]

Slogan from a public-service ad campaign for organ donation:
Some people need you inside them.   *— Kimberly Hefner, Former Playboy Playmate* [154]

The reason I don't sign the organ-donor part of my driver's license is that I can imagine an accident where I'm badly injured and a very large cop is standing over me whose uncle needs a kidney.   *— Lou Schneider* [196]

~ Treatment ~

Phineagle's Law: The more complicated one makes a treatment, the more hopelessly it will become botched. [201]

If you don't know how to treat something, change the diagnosis.

— W.B. Shelley, MD [135]

You can't make an asymptomatic patient better.   — *Anonymous* [94]

His indecision is final.   — *Anonymous* [135]

You don't have to be a schizophrenic to treat a schizophrenic.   — *Anonymous* [94]

When I was younger, if any of us kids got sick, my mother would bring out the chicken soup. Of course, that didn't work for broken bones. For broken bones, she gave us boiled beef.   — *George Burns* [242]

Here lie the bones of Susan Lowder
Who burst while drinking a Seidlitz powder.
Now she's gone to her Heavenly rest,
She should have waited till it effervesced.   — *Anonymous* [135]

A fellow went to his doctor because he wasn't feeling well.
   "Do you smoke excessively?" asked the doctor.
   "No."
   "Drink a lot?"
   "No."
   "Keep late hours?"
   "Nope."
   The doctor shook his head and said, "How can I cure you if you have nothing to give up?"

(See also Advice, Complications, Procedures)

~ TURFING ~

It is better to have turfed and lost than never to have turfed at all.
                                                                   — *Anonymous* [135]

When all else fails, turf the patient.   — *Anonymous* [94]

(See also Roundsmanship)

~ TV Doctors ~

I hope that people aren't watching TV News Doctors to stay healthy. Watching News Doctors to stay healthy is like watching "Star Trek" to become a better astronaut, although in all fairness some episodes of "Star Trek" are pretty realistic compared to TV news. — *Mark DePaolis, MD* [108]

Damn it, Jim, I'm a doctor not a bricklayer! — *Leonard "Bones" McCoy, MD* [294]

Compared to Ben Casey, Dr. Kildare is a placebo. — *Constance Rizzo* [258]

(See also Media)

𝒰

~ ULCERS ~

I don't have ulcers; I give them.

— Harry Cohn [103]

In the world of ulcers, Unger, you're what's known as a carrier.

— Dr. Gordon, "The Odd Couple" [233]

~ UMBILICAL CORD ~

The doctor took my baby out of my wife's belly. Then he turned to me and asked, "Mr. Goldthwait, would you like to cut the cord?" And I said, "Isn't there anyone more qualified?"

— Bobcat Goldthwait [67]

~ URINE ~

Some bring their sample in a jar,
Some bring it in a pot,
Some bring a sample hardly ample,
While others bring a lot.

— Richard Armour, Ph.D. [14]

Urinalysis, n. Relating to the environment of a second person with respect to the lodgings of a third person; as "I'm in Mary's room and urinalysis."

— H. S. Grannatt [145]

A few months ago, I read a study about the behavior of men in public bathrooms. It turns out that it takes the average man 8 seconds to pee after he stands in front of a urinal. However, if another man comes into the bathroom, it takes an extra 5 seconds before the man begins to go. In fact, the closer anyone comes to this *average* man, the longer it takes for him to do his business. Now, *that* was a study that needed to be done.

— Larry Bauer, MD [246]

I was having breakfast in the hospital, when a nurse came in with a specimen bottle. When she wasn't looking, I took my apple juice, poured it into the bottle, and handed it to her. She looked at the bottle and said, "My, we're looking a little cloudy today, aren't we?"—whereupon I took a big swig from the bottle and replied, "By George, you're right. Let's run it through again!"

— *Norman Cousins* [261]

On reaching old age:
First you forget names, then you forget faces; then you forget to pull your zipper up, then you forget to pull your zipper down.   — *Leo Rosenberg* [247]

An elderly woman goes to the doctor's office with a beautiful butterfly, mounted under glass, and presents it to the nurse. The nurse says, "This is very nice, Mrs. Brown, but it's not the type of specimen we had in mind."

~ UROLOGY ~

I don't need you to remind me of my age, I have a bladder to do that for me.

— *Stephen Fry* [133]

We're pretty strict about sleep habits in my house. The only thing that's allowed to wake me up at 5AM is my bladder.   — *Howard Bennett, MD* [48]

Urology Definitions:
• Testes: What you order when you don't know what a patient has.
• Urinate: What a nurse might say if a patient asks what room he's in.

Bloopers & Malapropisms:
• When you pin him down, he has some slowing of the stream.
• Dr. Marx is watching his prostate.
• The patient has a long history of stress *incompetence*. (incontinence)
• He was examined by a physician with a history of renal colic.
• The urine culture grew greater than 10^5 *orgasms*. (organisms)
• The patient requested a screen for *prosthetic* cancer. (prostatic)
• There was no residual seen after voiding on the upright film.
• Genital exam reveals that the patient is *circus sized*. (circumcised)

- Mr. Watson is a 46-year-old man whose chief complaint is a rash on his *grand* penis. (glans)
- The patient presented with a temperature of 102° and *fowl* smelling urine. (foul)
- The patient is living with a Foley catheter.

Randy Plotkin, a world-renowned urologist and expert on sexual dysfunction, was asked by a women's group to give a lecture on his specialty. Giving his standard talk about sex was an easy request to fill, but he decided to give a lecture on sailing instead.

The doctor knew very little about sailing, but promised himself to take time out from his busy schedule to learn about the sport. He went to the library to read about sailing and borrowed videotapes on sailing races. But when he arrived at the auditorium to give his talk, Plotkin felt a moment of panic about lecturing on a subject he still knew very little about. So instead, he gave his usual talk about sexual intercourse. The women were thrilled and applauded him wildly.

That afternoon, one of the women in the audience ran into the doctor's wife and gushed about what a wonderful speech he had given. "You must be very proud, Mrs. Plotkin. Your husband is such a good speaker and is so knowledgeable about his subject."

Mrs. Plotkin was taken aback. "Knowledgeable? He's only done it twice. Once he got sick and the other time his hat blew off!"

A man was running late for an appointment with a urologist. When he got to the medical building, he inadvertently walked into a podiatrist's office instead of the urologist.

"Sorry I'm late," the man said to the receptionist.

"I can't seem to find your chart, Mr. Patton," she said. "Why don't you have a seat in room 12 and the doctor will be right with you."

The patient took a seat and after a few minutes, the podiatrist entered the room.

"Let's have a look," the doctor said.

Mr. Patton unzipped his trousers and proceeded to show the doctor his problem.

"That's not a foot!" the podiatrist said.

"I didn't know there was a minimum requirement," the patient replied.

An old man goes to see a urologist complaining that he can't pee.

"How old are you?" the urologist asks.

"I'm 89-years-old," the man replies.

"Well," the urologist answers, "You've peed enough."

How many urologists does it take to change a light bulb?
—Five. One to screw it in and four to stand around cracking jokes about the old bulb.

(See also Circumcision, Impotence, Penis, Prostate Gland, Urinary Tract Infections)

~ UTERUS ~

It bugs me when a husband thinks his wife knows where everything is. Like he thinks the uterus is a tracking device. He comes in and says, "Hey, Roseanne! Roseanne! Do we have any Cheetos left?" Like he can't go over and lift up a sofa cushion himself.
— *Roseanne Barr* [23]

(See also Gynecology, Obstetrics)

$\mathcal{V}$

~ VACATIONS ~

One of my friends made a mistake on his last vacation. He inadvertently paid for room service with a credit card that had his "MD" printed on it. For the rest of his vacation, instead of finding little chocolate mints on his pillow at night, there were notes from the maid about her bursitis and the ailments of her 50-odd relatives.   — *Howard Bennett, MD* [38]

~ VAGINA ~

Aren't you a little old to be looking up words like this?
                                          — *George Thomas, MD & Lee Schreiner, MD* [303]

I was watching TV the other day when I saw this actress in a tampon commercial. Later that day, I saw the same actress in a douche commercial. So I thought to myself, lady I know way too much about your vagina.   — *Margaret Cho* [135]

~ VA HOSPITALS ~

There is no such thing as bowel function at the VA.   — *Anonymous* [94]

There are two goals for every patient who's admitted to a VA hospital. One is to keep the patient alive. The other is to make sure someone else does the discharge summary.   — *Howard Bennett, MD* [40]

~ VARICOSE VEINS ~

Varicose veins are the result of the improper selection of grandparents.
                                              — *William Osler, MD* [27]

~ VASECTOMY ~

A vasectomy means never having to say you're sorry.   *— Larry Adler* [103]

After a 40-year-old businessman had his annual physical, his doctor came out and said, "You had a great checkup. Is there anything else you'd like to talk about?"

"Well," the man said. "I was thinking about getting a vasectomy."

"That's a big decision," the doctor said. "Have you talked about it with your family?"

"Yes," the man said, "they're if favor of it 12 to 4."

A man goes to the hospital for a vasectomy. Shortly after he wakes up from the anesthesia, his urologist comes in and says, "Well, Bill, I've got some good news and some bad news."

"What's the bad news?" the patient says.

"I'm afraid we accidentally cut off your testicles during the procedure."

"Oh my God," the patient says, "What's the good news?"

"We had them biopsied and their not malignant."

(See also Birth Control)

~ VEGETARIANS ~

I am not a complete vegetarian. I only eat animals that have died in their sleep.
       — George Carlin [307]

Save a cow, eat a vegetarian.   *— Bumper sticker* [135]

A vegetarian is a person who won't eat anything that can have children.
       — David Brenner [135]

Never order anything in a vegetarian restaurant that would ordinarily have meat in it.   *— Tom Parker* [76]

To me, vegetables are not a food; they're an accessory. — *Gene Perret* [244]

Vegetables are interesting but lack a sense of purpose when unaccompanied by a good cut of meat. — *Fran Lebowitz* [190]

I did not rise to the top of the food chain to become a vegetarian. — *Bumper sticker* [135]

(See also Food, Health Food)

~ VENEREAL DISEASE ~

There was a young lady at sea
Who complained that it hurt her to pee.
   Said the brawny old mate,
   "That accounts for the state
Of the cook and the captain and me." — *Anonymous* [73]

Two elderly sisters go to see a new doctor. The doctor is a very thorough historian and asks the first one if she ever had gonorrhea. She says, "I don't know, let me ask my sister." The woman sticks her head in the next exam room and says, "Martha, have I ever had gonorrhea?" Her sister yells back, "I don't know, but if Medicare pays for it, get two!"

Pensky sat in his doctor's office. "I have a friend who's got venereal disease and he wants to know if it's difficult to cure."
   "It can be done," the doctor said.
   "Uh, my friend would like to know if it's expensive."
   "Not really," the doctor said. "If the case is advanced, the fee can be adjusted to match the patient's ability to pay."
   "One other thing," Pensky said. "My friend would like to know if the treatment hurts."
   "I don't know," the doctor said. "Take out your friend's penis and we'll see."

A 16-year-old went to the ER because of a penile discharge and painful urination. He filled out the requisite forms listing his age and address, etc. Under the space that said, "Responsible Party," he wrote, "My girlfriend."

~ VENIPUNCTURE ~

(See Blood & Blood Drawing)

~ VIRUS ~

Virus is a Latin word which, when used by doctors, translates to "Your guess is as good as mine."
— *Anonymous* [168]

My computer caught a health care virus. It goes through your system for hours, finds nothing wrong, and sends you a bill for $2,500.
— *Anonymous* [135]

There's always a virus going around.
— *Anonymous* [94]

~ VITAMINS ~

I tried Flintstones vitamins. I didn't feel any better, but I could stop the car with my feet.
— *Joan St. Onge* [88]

~ VOMITING ~

Paul's Axiom on the Conservation of Matter:
The amount of emesis will always exceed the capacity of the container provided for it. [101]

Nausea, n. Sensation experienced while the body decides whether to throw up or just die.
— *George Thomas, MD & Lee Scheiner, MD* [303]

A sensitive girl named O'Neill
Went up in a big Ferris Wheel;
   But when half-way around
   She looked down at the ground,
And it cost her a two-dollar meal.
— *Anonymous* [308]

Every authority on etiquette discusses how to put things into your stomach, but very few discuss how to get them back out in a hurry. Actually, there is no way to make vomiting courteous. You have to do the next best thing, which is to vomit is such a way that the story you tell about it later will be amusing.
— *P.J. O'Rourke* [235]

Frank Burns: Margaret, I should warn you that alcohol is quite fattening.
Hot Lips Houlihan: That's alright Frank, I plan on throwing up later.
— *"M*A*S*H"* [200]

~ WAITING ROOM ~

I'm fond of telling patients who I've kept waiting for more than sixty minutes, "About twenty years ago, I got two hours behind and I haven't quite caught up yet." My patients are not as fond of this story as I am.   — *Oscar London, MD* [192]

There are 332,000 doctors in the US and 205 million people. By long division it turns out that there is one doctor for every 617 people. Those are the 617 people you find ahead of you, waiting in your doctor's office.   — *Goodman Ace* [1]

There are two types of services in our society—those that require an appointment and those where you wait in line. Then there are doctor's visits, where you get to do both.   — *Howard Bennett, MD* [40]

Sign in a waiting room:
To avoid delay, have all of your symptoms ready. [135]

Over a lifetime, the average American spends 5 years waiting in lines, 2 years returning phone calls to people who aren't there, 1 year searching for misplaced objects, 8 months opening junk mail, and 6 months sitting at traffic lights—a total of more than 9 years. So what's another 30 minutes waiting to see the doctor?   — *Michael Fortinum* [129]

A 4-year-old boy is waiting to see the doctor for a sore throat. After an hour sitting around and reading books, the boy says to his mom, "Mommy, what's a cheetah?"
　　"It's a wild animal that lives in the jungle."
　　"What's a jungle?"
　　"It's part of the outdoors."
　　"What's outdoors?"
　　"Outside of this building."
　　"Will I ever go outdoors?"
　　The woman sighed, "I don't think so, dear."

An elderly man who had been sitting in the waiting room for a long time finally got up and said, "I think I'll go home and die a natural death."

"Sorry for the long wait," the doctor said to his last patient.

"That's okay," the patient said, "but it might have been nice to treat my illness in its early stages."

~ Ward Clerks ~

Ward clerk, n. The hospital's version of the appendix—every ward has one, but it's not clear what they do.   — *Howard Bennett, MD* (46)

Company clerking is hell. You're just doctors, you don't know the meaning of pressure.   — *Corporal Max Klinger, "M*A*S*H"* (200)

How many ward clerks does it take to change a light bulb?

— Three. Two to ignore your requests and one to hand you a requisition slip.

~ Wellness ~

A well person is a patient who has not been completely worked up.

— *J. Freymann, MD* (132)

Early to rise and early to bed makes a male healthy and wealthy and dead.

— *James Thurber* (125)

The human body is like a condominium. The thing that keeps you from really enjoying it is the maintenance.   — *Jerry Seinfeld* (275)

Obsession is no longer a disease, but an essential attribute of staying healthy.

— *Clifton Meador, MD* (209)

The average healthy, well-adjusted adult gets up at 7:30 in the morning feeling just plain terrible.   — *Jean Kerr* (172)

In the past 20 years the compendium of fatal foods has, at one time or another, included everything consumed by the human race. The only way to live forever, it seems, is never to eat again. — *Russel Baker* [21]

(See also Exercise, Health, Self-Help)

~ WRITING & PUBLISHING ~

The only thing doctors do more than write is procrastinate about writing.
— *Anonymous* [43]

On writing titles for articles:
Titles are best written with a brandy after dinner. Titles written on an empty stomach are likely to be dull and witless.   — *Berril Yushomerski Yankelowitz, MD* [324]

On getting two or more publications out of the same research:
In this day when fame and academic promotion depend on the dry weight of a curriculum vitae rather that its content, it is important to get as much out of a piece of work as one can.   — *Berril Yushomerski Yankelowitz, MD* [324]

On writing guides for doctors:
These guides seem to be composed by well-meaning people with the word-bound neurons of a constipated hippopotamus.   — *Anonymous* [212]

It's fun to write introductions—one is not constrained by facts.
— *Harry F. Harlow, Ph.D.* [152]

On fears of using too many references in a paper:
The author should remember that he is not reading the literature—just citing it.
— *Harry F. Harlow, Ph.D.* [152]

How many editors does it take to change a light bulb?
—Two. One to screw it in and one to send a rejection letter to the old bulb.

(See also Academia, Case Reports, Tenure)

X-Y-Z

~ X-RAYS ~

The attending physician put a patient's x-ray on the view box and turned to the medical student beside him.

"As you can see, one of the patient's legs is two inches shorter than the other because of a deformed tibia. This causes the patient to limp. Now, what would you do in a case like this?"

"Well, doctor," the student said. "I guess I'd limp too."

"You seem to be recovering nicely," the doctor said. "These x-rays show some damage to the bone, but I wouldn't worry about it."

The patient said, "If your bones were damaged, I wouldn't worry about it either."

A 5-year-old girl needed an x-ray to see if she broke her arm. When she came out of the x-ray room, she told her mother, "They took a picture of my bones, mom."

"Yes, dear," her mother replied. "Did everything go all right?"

"Sure," said the girl. "It was amazing. I didn't even have to take my skin off."

(See also Radiology)

~ YOUTH ~

Youth is that period when a young boy knows everything but how to make a living.
— *Carey McWilliams* [197]

Youth is a disease from which we all recover.
— *Dorothy Parker* [67]

Youth is a wonderful thing. What a crime to waste it on children.

— *George Bernard Shaw* [93]

(See also Children)

~ Zoonoses ~

Even though animals can transmit diseases to people, they also give them a lot of happiness, which probably balances things out in the long run. People may catch diseases, but at least they die happier.

— *Alan Ayckbourn* [18]

References

Most of the references are listed in the standard way. In a few cases, you will notice the letter "A" before a page number. This indicates that the material was published in a journal's advertising pages.

1. Ace G: Top of my head. Saturday Review, September 1964.
2. Adams, Joey: Joey Adams' Complete Encyclopedia of Laughter. West Hollywood, CA: Dove Books, 1996.
3. Adelman, S: Nanny Tyrannica. In, Nancy Davis (ed), Creme de la Femme. New York: Random House, 1997.
4. Allen, Woody: Play It Again Sam. New York: Random House, 1969.
5. Allen, Woody, and Marshall Brickman: Sleeper (screenplay), 1973.
6. Allen, Woody: Love and Death (screenplay), 1975.
7. Allen, Woody: Death (A Play). In, Without Feathers. New York: Random House, 1975.
8. Allen, Woody: Quoted in the New York Times, December 1975.
9. Allen, Woody, and Marshall Brickman: Annie Hall (screenplay), 1977.
10. Allen, Woody: Crimes and Misdemeanors (screenplay), 1989.
11. Alpern, Lynne, and Esther Blumenthal: Oh, Lord, I Sound Just Like Mama, 1986.
12. Applewhite, Ashton, William R. Evans, and Andrew Frothingham: And I Quote. New York: St. Martin's Press, 1992.
13. Armor, Joyce: The Dictionary According to Mommy. New York: Meadowbrook Press, 1989.
14. Armour R: Urinalysis. Postgraduate Medicine 1959;26(10):A252.
15. Armstrong N: Quoted in the Guinness Book of Sports Quotations, 1990.
16. Asquith, Margaret: The Autobiography of Margaret Asquith, 1923.
17. Astor, N: Quoted in Reader's Digest, 1960.
18. Ayckbourn, Alan: Woman in Mind, 1986.
19. Ayres, Alex: The Wit & Wisdom of Mark Twain. New York: Harper & Row, 1987.
20. Ayres, Alex: The Wit and Wisdom of Will Rogers. New York: Meridian Books, 1993.
21. Baker, Russell: The Rescue of Miss Yaskell and Other Pipe Dreams. New York: Congdon & Weed, Inc., 1983.
22. Barreca, Regina: The Penguin Book of Women's Humor. New York: Penguin Books, 1996.
23. Barreca, Regina: The Signet Book of American Humor. New York: Signet, 1999.
24. Barry, Dave: Bad Habits. New York: Henry Holt and Company, 1987.
25. Barry, Dave: Dave Barry Talks Back. New York: Crown Publishers, 1991.
26. Barry, Dave: Dave Barry is from Mars and Venus. New York: Ballantine Books, 1997.
27. Bean, William Bennett: Sir William Osler's Aphorisms: From His Bedside Teachings and Writings. New York: Henry Schuman, Inc., 1950.
28. Bean, William Bennett: Rare Diseases and Lesions. Springfield: Charles C. Thomas, 1967.
29. Behrman, Sid: The Doctor Joke Book. New York: Barnes & Noble Books, 1995.
30. Belloc, Hilaire: Henry King, 1907.
31. Bennett, Alan: Habeas Corpus, 1973.
32. Bennett HJ: How to survive a case presentation. Chest 1985;88:292–294.
33. Bennett HJ: The student's dilemma. Postgraduate Medicine 1986;80(5):266–274.
34. Bennett HJ: The teething virus. Pediatric Infectious Disease Journal 1986;5: 399–401.
35. Bennett HJ: The pediatric internship screening test. Contemporary Pediatrics 1987;4(5):96–99.
36. Bennett HJ: Letters to the editor that I'd like to see. Resident & Staff Physician 1992; 38(7):72–74.

37. Bennett HJ: A guide for interpreting what academic specialists really mean. Journal of Family Practice 1992;34:505–507.
38. Bennett HJ: How to survive your next vacation. Postgraduate Medicine 1992;91(6):49–53.
39. Bennett HJ: Health care reform or bust. Journal of Family Practice 1994;39:393–394.
40. Bennett HJ: A CAT scan a day keeps the lawyers away: rules and observations for the '90s. Journal of Family Practice 1994;39:421–422.
41. Bennett HJ: Nighttime rhymes. Journal of Family Practice 1995;41:535.
42. Bennett HJ: Top ten lists for doctors—part II. Journal of Family Practice 1996;43:110.
43. Bennett, Howard J: The Best of Medical Humor: A Collection of Articles, Essays, Poetry & Letters Published in the Medical Literature. Philadelphia: Hanley & Belfus, 2nd edition, 1997.
44. Bennett HJ: Night call is for the birds. Journal of Family Practice 1997;45:187–188.
45. Bennett HJ: Mother Goose, MD. Stitches 1998;July:32–34.
46. Bennett HJ: The doctor's dictionary. Journal of Family Practice 1999;48:313.
47. Bennett HJ: Medicated nursery rhymes. Obstetrics & Gynecology, in press.
48. Bennett HJ: Unpublished material used in lectures or written for the collection.
49. Bennett JH: You know you're a physician executive if…. Journal of Family Practice 1997; 45:281–284.
50. Bessman SP: Yoo-yoo. New England Journal of Medicine 1965;273:651.
51. Bierce, Ambrose: The Devil's Dictionary, 1911.
52. Bigwood M: JAMA 1962;181(2):A264.
53. Billings JS: On vital and medical statistics. Medical Record 1889;36(22):589.
54. Black, Laura: Strathgallant, 1981.
55. Blake, E: Quoted in the Observer, February 1983.
56. Bluestone N: Who says doctors can't write? Pennsylvania Medicine 1983;86(11):48.
57. "The Bob Newhart Show" (television series), 1972–1978.
58. Bombeck, Erma, with Bil Keane: Just Wait Till You Have Children of Your Own, 1971.
59. Boren JH: Arcane and proud of it. New York Times, June 4, 1998.
60. Bornemeier, WC: Sphincter protecting hemorrhoidectomy. American Journal of Proctology 1960;11:48–52.
61. Bosker, Gideon: Medicine is the Best Laughter. St. Louis: Mosby, 1995.
62. Brallier, Jess M: Medical Wit & Wisdom. Philadelphia: Running Press, 1993.
63. Brancati F: The art of pimping. JAMA 1989;262:89–90.
64. Brancati F: Readers of the lost chart: an archaeological approach to the medical record. JAMA 1992;267:1860–1861.
65. Braude, Jacob M: Braude's Treasury of Wit & Humor for all Occasions. Englewood Cliffs, NJ: Prentice Hall, 1991.
66. Brilliant, Ashleigh: We've Been Through So Much Together, and Most of It Was Your Fault. Santa Barbara, CA: Woodbridge Press Publishing Co., 1999.
67. Brown, Judy: Joke Soup. Kansas City: Andrews McMeel Publishing, 1998.
68. Brown, Michelle, and Ann O'Connor: Hammer & Tongues: The Best of Women's Wit and Humor. New York: McGraw-Hill, 1986.
69. Brown, Rita Mae: Starting from Scratch, 1988.
70. Brunton S: Quoted in Medical World News 1988;29(3):62.
71. Brussel, Eugene E: Webster's New World Dictionary of Quotable Definitions. Englewood Cliffs, NJ: Prentice Hall, 1988.
72. Buckley, Christopher: Wry Martinis. New York: Random House, 1997.
73. Butterfield WC: Know any bawdy old medical limericks? Medical Economics 1973;50(Jan 8):166.
74. Byrne, Robert: 1,911 Best Things Anybody Ever Said. New York: Fawcett Crest, 1988.
75. Byrne, Robert: The Fourth and by Far the Most Recent 637 Best Things Anybody Ever Said. New York: Fawcett Crest, 1990.
76. Byrne, Robert: The Fifth and Far Funnier than the First Four 637 Best Things Anybody Ever Said. New York: Fawcett Crest, 1993.

77. Caen H: Quoted in Medical World News 1988;29(7):90.
78. Caen H: Quoted in Medical World News 1988;29(10):54.
79. Caen H: Quoted in Medical World News 1990;31(15):62.
80. Calhoun LG, et al: An overview of research findings in the behavioral sciences: the laws of psychology. Journal of Polymorphous Perversity 1987;4(1):3–4.
81. Caplan AN: The gout. New England Journal of Medicine 1966;275:664.
82. Carlton LE: Song to my plastic surgeon. JAMA 1961;178(1):A276.
83. Carleton R: Quoted in Medical World News 1990;31(3):68.
84. Carter, Judy: Stand-up Comedy: The Book. New York: Dell Publishing, 1989.
85. Cerf, Bennett: Out On A Limerick. New York: Harper & Row, 1960.
86. Chayefsky, Paddy: The Hospital (screenplay). Simcha Productions, 1971.
87. "Cheers" (television series), 1982–1993.
88. Christing, Adam: Comedy Comes Clean. New York: Crown Trade Paperbacks, 1996.
89. Christing, Adam: Comedy Comes Clean-2. New York: Crown Trade Paperbacks, 1997.
90. City Slickers (screenplay), 1991.
91. City Slickers II (screenplay), 1994.
92. Clark, Steven E: Steel Magnolias (screenplay), 1989.
93. Claro, Joe: Random House Book of Jokes and Anecdotes. New York: Random House, 1996.
94. Classic Medical Quote: No source available.
95. Cohen M: Quoted in Medical World News 1988;29(5):100.
96. Cohl, H. Aaron: The Friar's Club Encyclopedia of Jokes. New York: Black Dog & Levanthal Publishers, 1997.
97. Conti R: Quoted in Medical World News 1990;31(9):44.
98. Cowan, Lore, and Maurice Cowan: The Wit of Women. London: Leslie Frewin Ltd., 1969.
99. Cowan, Lore, and Maurice Cowan: The Wit of Medicine. London: Leslie Frewin Ltd., 1972.
100. Cox, Marcelene: Quoted in Ladies' Home Journal, 1945.
101. Curry J: Official explanations of emergency nursing. Journal of Emergency Nursing 1991;17(2):120–122.
102. Da Costa, J. Chalmers: The Trials and Triumphs of the Surgeon. Philadelphia: Dorrance, 1944.
103. Daintith, John, and Amanda Isaacs: Medical Quotes: A Thematic Dictionary. New York: Facts on File, 1989.
104. Davis, Eddie: Laugh Yourself Well. New York: Frederick Fell, Inc., 1954.
105. DeFord, Deborah: Quotable Quotes. Pleasantville, NY: Reader's Digest Association, 1997.
106. DeFord, Deborah: Laughter, the Best Medicine. Pleasantville, NY: Reader's Digest Association, 1997.
107. DePaolis M: Conference call. Postgraduate Medicine 1993;93(5):57–58.
108. DePaolis, Mark: "Trust Me, I'm a Doctor." Minneapolis: Fairview Press, 1995.
109. DePaolis, Mark: Are You a Real Doctor? Minneapolis: Fairview Press, 1997.
110. DePaolis, Mark: Get Well Sooner. Minneapolis: Fairview Press, 1997.
111. Dickson P: Life's little rules. Washingtonian, October 1999.
112. Diller, Phyllis: The Joys of Aging and How to Avoid Them, 1981.
113. Dimmick EL: Hamlet's soliloquy on allergy. Obstetrics & Gynecology 1962;20:148.
114. Dolezal J, Pamondon J: Translating medical idiom. New England Journal of Medicine 1976;295:176.
115. Dowden J: Getting to the bottom of it all. In, Hawkins, Clifford (ed): Alimentary My Dear Doctor. Oxford: Radcliffe Medical Press, 1988.
116. Drennan, Robert E: The Algonquin Wits. New York: Citadel Press, 1995.
117. Durst W: Quoted in Medical World News 1988;29(24):62.
118. Einstein A: Quoted in Time Magazine, December 1999.
119. Elders J: Quoted in Medical World News 1993;34(10):52.
120. Ellis R, Lancaster DJ: Cephawhatchamacallums. New England Journal of Medicine 1989;320:872.

121. English, Horace B., and Ava C. English: A Comprehensive Dictionary of Psychological and Psychoanalytic Terms, 1958.
122. Ephron, Delia: Funny Sauce. New York: Viking, 1986.
123. Ephron, Nora: When Harry Met Sally (screenplay), 1989.
124. Esar, Evan: 20,000 Quips & Quotes, 1968.
125. Fabricant, Noah D: Amusing Quotations for Doctors and Patients. New York: Grune & Stratton, 1950.
126. Feinstein A: Quoted in Medical World News 1991;32(11):44.
127. Fitzgerald FT: A doctor's glossary. The Pharos 1982(Winter):18.
128. Fleming A: Quoted in Medical World News 1989;29(8):114.
129. Fortinum M: Quoted in Medical World News 1988;29(14):56.
130. Fraser AG, et al: The haggis tolerance test in Scots and Sassenachs. British Medical Journal 1988;297:1632–1634.
131. "Frasier" (television series), 1993–present.
132. Freymann J: Quoted in, Meador C: The last well person. New England Journal of Medicine 1994;330:440–441.
133. Fry, Stephen: Paperweight, 1992.
134. Fuchs, Ronald D: You Said a Mouthful: Wise and Witty Quotations About Food. New York: St. Martin's Press, 1996.
135. Funny quote or one-liner found on TV, the internet, or sent in by a colleague: No source available.
136. Gaño, SN: A gloss attributed to the Hippocratic school. The Leech 1958;4(8):17–19.
137. Garden, Graeme: The Best Medicine. New York: St. Martin's Press, 1984.
138. Garrison FH: Medical proverbs, aphorisms and epigrams. Bulletin of the New York Academy of Medicine 1928;4:979–1005.
139. Gold, Todd: Comic Relief. New York: Avon Books, 1996.
140. Goldblatt D: Off to the yearly convention. New England Journal of Medicine 1974; 290:1385.
141. Golden, Francis L: For Doctors Only. New York: Frederick Fell, Inc., 1948.
142. Golden, Francis L: Jest What the Doctor Ordered. New York: Frederick Fell, Inc., 1949.
143. Gordon, Leo A: Gordon's Guide to the Surgical Morbidity and Mortality Conference. Philadelphia: Hanley & Belfus, 1994.
144. Grannatt HS: Notes from a medical lexicographer's waste basket. JAMA 176(8):A236.
145. Grannatt HS: Notes from a medical lexicographer's waste basket. JAMA 178(3):A246.
146. Greenberg D: Grant Swinger's innovations. New England Journal of Medicine 1977; 297:459–460.
147. Greer, Germaine: The Female Eunuch, 1970.
148. Grizzard, Lewis: The Wit and Wisdom of Lewis Grizzard. Atlanta: Longstreet Press, 1995.
149. Groening, Matt: Bart Simpson's Guide to Life. New York: Harperperennial, 1993.
150. Groening, Matt: Basic facts for today's young folk. In, Life in Hell, 1996.
151. Guttman D: Things they never warned me about in medical school. Medical Economics 1985;62(Dec 23):59.
152. Harlow HF: Fundamental principles for preparing psychology journal articles. Anesthesia and Analgesia 1976;55:455–458.
153. Hayes, John H: From Bed to Verse. Chicago: Physician's Record Company, 1958.
154. Hefner K: Quoted in Physician's Weekly, December 1995.
155. Hennekens C: Remark heard at a medical conference, 1998.
156. Herscovitch J: Ethical principles of psychologists: an update. Journal of Polymorphous Perversity 1985;2(2):9.
157. Hess, Joan: A Really Cute Corpse, 1988.
158. Hipps, John G: The Country Doctor. Emporium, PA: Wonderworld, 1989.
159. Holmes, Oliver Wendell: Medical Essays. Boston: Houghton Mifflin, 1911.
160. "Honey, I Shrunk the Kids" (screenplay), 1989.

161. "The Honeymooners" (television series), 1955–1956.
162. Hopcraft, K: A gut feeling. In, Hawkins, Clifford (ed): Alimentary My Dear Doctor. Oxford: Radcliffe Medical Press, 1988.
163. Hudson, Lisa J., Genevieve Field, and Jake Morrissey: That's Funny. New York: Cader Books, 1996.
164. Hutter A: Quoted in Medical World News 1990;31(9):44.
165. Jacobson M: Quoted in Medical World News 1989;30(9):82.
166. JAMA 1963;183(12):A226. Published in "Smile A While" column.
167. JAMA 1997;278:1200. Quoted in a book review by Frederick L. Glauser.
168. Jarman, Colin: The Guinness Book of Poisonous Quotes. Chicago: Contemporary Books, 1993.
169. Johnson, Eric W: A Treasury of Humor. Buffalo, NY: Prometheus Books, 1989.
170. Joynt RJ: A note for interns and residents: a new law and advice on its circumvention. Perspectives in Biology and Medicine 1981;25:144–147.
171. Kannel W: Quoted in Medical World News 1990;31(15):44.
172. Kerr, Jean: Please Don't Eat the Daisies, 1957.
173. Kerr, Jean: Poor Richard, 1965
174. Kerr, Jean: The ten worst things about a man. McCall's, 1960.
175. Kessler D: Quoted in Medical World News. 1992;33(5):48.
176. Kilbourne PA: Short course in euphemism. Medical Economics 1963;40(Feb 25): 90–91.
177. Kindergarten Cop (screenplay), 1990.
178. Kitchen BG: Debunking the bunk. JAMA 1964;188(7):A234.
179. Klein, Allen: The Healing Power of Humor. Los Angeles: Jeremy P. Tarcher, Inc., 1989.
180. Klein, Allen: Quotations to Cheer You Up When the World is Getting You Down. New York: Wings Books, 1991.
181. Knebel, Fletcher: Quoted in Reader's Digest, 1961.
182. LaCombe MA: At last! Blessed relief for the pain and discomfort of percentorrhea. Hospital Physician 1971;7(2):102–103.
183. Lamott, Anne: Operating Instructions. New York: Fawcett Columbine, 1993.
184. Lansky, Bruce: Age Happens. New York: Meadowbrook Press, 1996.
185. Lansky, Bruce: Familiarity Breeds Children. New York: Meadowbrook Press, 1997.
186. Lansky, Bruce: Laugh Twice and Call Me in the Morning. New York: Meadowbrook Press, 1999.
187. Latham E: Famous Sayings and Their Authors, 1904.
188. Lax, Eric: On Being Funny: Woody Allen and Comedy, 1975.
189. Lebowitz, Fran: Social Studies. In, The Fran Lebowitz Reader. New York: Vintage Books, 1994.
190. Lebowitz, Fran: Metropolitan Life. In, The Fran Lebowitz Reader. New York: Vintage Books, 1994.
191. Lieberman, Gerald F: 3,500 Good Quotes for Speakers. New York: Doubleday, 1983.
192. London, Oscar: Kill as Few Patients as Possible. Berkley: Ten Speed Press, 1987.
193. Mabry RL: There oughtta be a law. Southern Medical Journal 1988;81:1295–1296.
194. MacHale, Des: Wit. Boulder, CO: Roberts Rinehart Publishers, 1998.
195. Maggio, Rosalie: The New Beacon Book of Quotations by Women. Boston: Beacon Press, 1996.
196. Malloy, Merrit: Irish-American Funny Quotes. New York: Sterling Publishing, 1994.
197. Malloy, Merrit, and Marsha Rose: Comedians' Quote Book. New York: Sterling Publishing, 1993.
198. Markoe, Merrill: How to Be Hap-Hap-Happy Like Me. New York: Viking, 1994.
199. Martin, HB: The last of the detail men. JAMA 1961;177(1):A206–210.
200. "M*A*S*H" (television series), 1972–1983.
201. Matz R: Principles of medicine. New York State Journal of Medicine 1977;77:99–101
202. Matz R: More principles of medicine. New York State Journal of Medicine 1977;1984–1985.

203. Matz R: Still more principles of medicine. New York State Journal of Medicine 1980; 113–116.

204. "Maude" (television series), 1972–1978.

205. Maugham, W. Somerset: Of Human Bondage, 1915.

206. McCann, Sean: The Wit of Oscar Wilde. New York: Dorset Press, 1969.

207. McFadden ER: Quoted in Medical World News 1988;29(17):70.

208. McHugh P: Quoted in Medical World News 1990;31(15):62.

209. Meador C: The last well person. New England Journal of Medicine 1994;330:440–441.

210. Meador, Clifton K: A Little Book of Doctors' Rules II. Philadelphia: Hanley & Belfus, 1999.

211. Medical World News 1989;30(20):58. Quoted in Risus Column.

212. Medical World News 1990;30(19):76. Quoted in Risus Column.

213. Medical World News 1990;31(12):48. Quoted in Risus Column.

214. Medical World News 1991;32(5):65. Quoted in Risus Column.

215. Merken G: Quoted in Medical World News 1989;30(13):54.

216. Merrel SW, McGreevy JM: Surgical aphorisms. Western Journal of Medicine 1991;154: 110–111.

217. Metcalf, Fred: The Penguin Dictionary of Modern Humorous Quotations. New York: Viking, 1986.

218. Metcalf, Fred: The Penguin Dictionary of Jokes. New York: Viking, 1993.

219. Meyers, James E: A Treasury of Medical Humor. Springfield, IL: Lincoln-Herndon Press, 1993.

220. Midler, B: Quoted in Reader's Digest, 1982.

221. Miller, Dennis: Ranting Again. New York: Doubleday, 1998.

222. Mills JB: A patient looks at gastrointestinal endoscopy. Gastrointestinal Endoscopy 1986;32:304.

223. Mingo, Jack, and John Javna: Primetime Proverbs: The Book of TV Quotes. New York: Harmony Books, 1989.

224. Morgan C: Quoted in Medical World News 1989;30(16).

225. Mouchawar A: Quoted in Medical World News 1988;29(18):70.

226. Murphy C: Psychoanalysis: a layperson's guide to theory and technique. In, Glenn C. Ellenbogen (ed), The Primal Whimper. New York: The Guilford Press, 1989.

227. Nall JO: Vogues. JAMA 1967;200(5):A226.

228. Nash, Ogden: Bed Riddance: A Posy for the Indisposed. Boston: Little, Brown, 1970.

229. Nash, Ogden: Quoted in Lite Medicine 1996;1(1):8.

230. Neuman, Alfred E: Mad Magazine Symbol.

231. Newman TB, Browner WS: The epidemiology of life and death: a critical commentary. American Journal of Public Health 1988;78:161–162.

232. Novak, William, and Moshe Waldoks: The Big Book of New American Humor. New York: HarperPerennial, 1990.

233. "The Odd Couple" (television series), 1970–1975.

234. Orben, Robert: 2,000 Sure-Fire Jokes for Speakers. New York: Doubleday, 1986.

235. O'Rourke, PJ: Modern Manners. New York: Atlantic Monthly Press, 1989.

236. Osler W: Quoted in JAMA 1986;255:302.

237. Paretsky S: The case of the Pietro Andromache. In, Wallace Marilyn (ed): Sisters in Crime, 1989.

238. Parker Dorothy: Quoted in Vanity Fair, 1925.

239. Parker Dorothy: "Résumé." In, Enough Rope, 1926.

240. Parker Dorothy: Telegram sent to a friend. In, Meade, Marion: Dorothy Parker: What Fresh Hell is This?, 1988.

241. Parrott, EO: The Penguin Book of Limericks. New York: Penguin Books, 1984.

242. Perret, Gene: Classic One-Liners. New York: Sterling Publishing Co., 1994.

243. Perret, Gene: Hilarious One-Liners. New York: Sterling Publishing Co., 1996.

244. Perret, Gene: Great One-Liners. New York: Sterling Publishing Co., 1992.

245. Perret, Gene: Roasts & Toasts. New York: Sterling Publishing Co., 1997.

246. Personal Communication.

247. Peter, Laurence J: Peter's Quotations. New York: Quill, 1977.

248. Pfeiffer, Rip: A Chance to Cut is a Chance to Cure. Copyright 1983, Ralph B. Pfeiffer.

249. Phillips, Bob: Phillips' Book of Great Thoughts and Funny Sayings. Wheaton, IL: Tyndale House Publishers, 1993.

250. Poole, Mary Pettibone: A Glass Eye at a Keyhole, 1938.

251. Prochnow, Herbert V., and Herbert V. Prochnow, Jr: Dictionary of Wit, Wisdom & Satire. New York: Harper & Brothers, 1962.

252. Ramsey C: Quoted in Medical World News 1991;32(2):64.

253. Rebeta-Burditt, Joyce: The Cracker Factory, 1977.

254. Reichman L: Quoted in Medical World News 1988;29(19):126.

255. Ricks AE: Passing through third year—a guide for weary travelers. The New Physician 1982;31(8):16–19.

256. Ricks, Anne Eva: The Official MD Handbook. New York: Plume Books, 1983.

257. Ricks AE: Making the grade: how to evaluate medical students. Resident & Staff Physician 1985;31(6):65–66.

258. Rizzo C: A dictionary "twist." JAMA 1962;180(9):A216.

259. Robertson M: Quoted in Medical World News 1990;31(14):62.

260. Robbins, Stanley L., Ramzi S. Cotran, and Vinay Kumar: Pathologic Basis of Disease. Philadelphia: W.B. Saunders, 1984.

261. Robinson, Vera M: Humor and the Health Professions. Thorofare, NJ: Slack Inc., 1991.

262. Rogers, Will: The Illiterate Digest, 1924.

263. Rooney, Andy: Word for Word. New York: G.P. Putnam's Sons, 1986.

264. Rose I: Fellowshipmanship. Canadian Medical Association Journal 1962;87:1232–1235.

265. Rose I: The professional patient. Canadian Medical Association Journal 1965;92:923–926.

266. Rose I: Lectureshipmanship. Canadian Medical Association Journal 1969;101:114–116.

267. "Roseanne" (television series), 1988–1997.

268. Rosten, Leo: Leo Rosten's Carnival of Wit. New York: Dutton Books, 1994.

269. Rosten, Leo: Leo Rosten's Giant Book of Laughter. New York: Bonanza Books, 1985.

270. Rubin B: Cephalomalacia obfuscate. Pediatric Infectious Disease Journal 1983;2:424–425.

271. Rudner, Rita: Naked Beneath My Clothes. New York: Penguin Books, 1991.

272. Rumble CT: "The storm before the calm." Psychiatric Communications 1964;7:35–38.

273. Saretsky, Theodor: How to Make Your Analyst Love You. New York: Citadel Press, 1993.

274. Scott RS, Myles WM: Ophthalmic diction-err-y. Survey Ophthalmology 1994;38:570.

275. Seinfeld, Jerry: SeinLanguage. New York: Bantam Books, 1993.

276. "Seinfeld" (television series), 1990–1998.

277. Shaftner K: Mater Anser: nursery rhymes for physicians. Journal of Family Practice 1997;44:216.

278. Shaw A: Today's most "in" specialty. Medical Economics 1975;52(June 9):53.

279. Shaw, George Bernard: Back to Methuselah, 1921.

280. Sheiner LB: Quoted in Medical World News 1991;32(5):65.

281. Shem, Samuel: The House of God. New York: Dell Publishing, 1978.

282. Shem, Samuel: Fine. New York: St. Martin's Press, 1985.

283. Sherrin, Ned: The Oxford Dictionary of Humorous Quotations. New York: Oxford University Press, 1995.

284. Sherwin, Jill: Quotable Star Trek. New York: Pocket Books, 1999.

285. Shike M: Quoted in Medical World News 1991;32(8):52.

286. Simon, Neil: The Odd Couple, 1966.

287. Simon, Neil: The Gingerbread Lady, 1970.

288. Simon, Neil: Only When I Laugh (screenplay), 1981.

289. Smith, Elinor Goulding: The Complete Book of Absolutely Perfect Baby and Child Care. New York: Harcourt, Brace and Company, 1957.

290. Smith RP: Conference coma. Obstetrics & Gynecology 1983;61:647–648.

291. Spence, Wayman R: Perez on Medicine. Waco, TX: WRS Publishing, 1993.

292. Spitzer A: Spitzer's laws of neonatology. Clinical Pediatrics 1981;20:733.

293. Spock B: Quoted in Bartlett's Unfamiliar Quotations, 1971.

294. "Star Trek" (The Original Series), 1966–1969.

295. "Star Trek" (The Next Generation), 1987–1994.

296. Steinem, Gloria: If Men Could Menstruate. In, Outrageous Acts and Everyday Rebellions. New York: Henry Holt and Company, 1983.

297. Stewart MM: Practical anatomy. JAMA 1968:204(4):A148.

298. Strauss, Maurice B: Familiar Medical Quotations. Boston: Little, Brown and Company, 1968.

299. Sullivan L: Quoted in Medical World News 1992;33(3):64.

300. Swenson P: Communicating with surgeons, once you learn the language, is possible most of the time. AORN Journal 1984;40:784–785.

301. Taylor PJ: The no-show patient never has the last appointment of the day. Canadian Medical Association Journal 1991;144:916.

302. Telesco M: Telesco's laws. American Journal of Nursing 1978;78:168.

303. Thomas, George, and Lee Schreiner: That's Incurable. New York: Penguin Books, 1984.

304. Thomas, Lewis: The Lives of a Cell. New York: Viking Press, 1974.

305. Thompson EM: All creatures, great and small. Journal of Family Practice 1998;47:155–156.

306. Twain, Mark: Quoted in Reader's Digest, 1939.

307. Uncle John's Legendary Lost Bathroom Reader. Ashland, Oregon: Bathroom Reader's Press, 1999.

308. Untermeyer, Louis: Lots of Limericks. New York: Barnes & Noble Books, 1961.

309. Wagner J: Quoted in Ms. Magazine, 1990.

310. Warren, Roz (ed.): Glibquips. Freedom, CA: The Crossing Press, 1994.

311. Warren, Roz (ed): Women's Lip. Naperville, IL: Hysteria Publications, 1998.

312. Waters, Daniel James: A Surgeon's Little Instruction Book. St. Louis: Quality Medical Publishing, 1998.

313. Welch WH: Twenty-fifth anniversary of the Johns Hopkins Hospital, 1889–1914. Johns Hopkins Hospital Bulletin 1914;25:363–366.

314. White, E.B., and Katharine S. White: A Subtreasury of American Humor. New York: Coward-McCann, Inc., 1941.

315. White, EB: Quoted in Harper's Magazine, November 1941.

316. Wilde, Larry: The Official Doctor's Joke Book. New York: Bantam Books, 1987.

317. Wilde, Oscar: A Woman of No Importance, 1893.

318. Wilde, Oscar: An Ideal Husband, 1895.

319. Winik, Marion: The Lunch-Box Chronicles. New York: Pantheon Books, 1998.

320. Winokur, Jon: The Portable Curmudgeon. New York: Plume Books, 1987.

321. Winokur, Jon: Friendly Advice. New York: Plume Books, 1990.

322. Winokur, Jon: Return of The Portable Curmudgeon. New York: Plume Books, 1992.

323. Wooten, Patty: Heart, Humor, & Healing. Mount Shasta, CA: Commune-A-Key Publishing, 1994.

324. Yankelowitz BY: How to write nifty titles for your papers. British Medical Journal 1980;1:96.

Index

Since the book is organized alphabetically, the index is primarily for author's names. The following subjects are included, however, because it should help with the retrieval of this material: Bloopers & Malapropisms, Limericks, Movies, Rules, Laws, & Axioms, Specialty Definitions, Television Shows, and Verse.

*Friend of Author